Doctors Look at Macrobiotics

Doctors Look at
Macrobiotics

Foreword by Lawrence H. Kushi, Sc.D.
Introduction by Michio Kushi

With Special Contributions by

Vivien Newbold, M.D.
Martha Cottrell, M.D.
Henry E. Altenberg, M.D.
Stephen Harnish, M.D.
Helen V. Farrell, M.D.

Christiane Northrup, M.D.
Marc Van Cauwenberghe, M.D.
David Dodson, M.D.
Guillermo Asis, M.D.
Terry Shintani, M.D.

Edited by Edward Esko

Japan Publications, Inc.

Note to the reader: Those with health problems are advised to seek the guidance of a qualified medical or psychological professional in addition to a qualified macrobiotic counselor before implementing any of the dietary and other approaches presented in this book. It is essential that any readers who have any reason to suspect serious illness in themselves or their family members seek appropriate medical, nutritional, or psychological advice promptly. Neither this or any other health related book should be used as a substitute for qualified care or treatment.

Published by JAPAN PUBLICATIONS, INC., Tokyo and New York

Distributors:
UNITED STATES: *Kodansha International/USA, Ltd., through Harper & Row, Publishers, Inc., 10 East 53rd Street, New York, New York 10022.* CANADA: *Fitzhenry & Whiteside Ltd., 195 Allstate Parkway, Markham, Ontario, L3R 4T8.* MEXICO AND CENTRAL AMERICA: *HARLA S. A. de C. V., Apartado 30-546, Mexico 4, D. F.* BRITISH ISLES: *Premier Book Marketing Ltd., 1 Gower Street, London WC1E 6HA.* EUROPEAN CONTINENT: *European Book Service PBD Strijkviertel 63, 3454 PK de Meern, The Netherlands.* AUSTRALIA AND NEW ZEALAND: *Bookwise International, 1 Jeanes Street, Beverley, South Australia 5007.* THE FAR EAST AND JAPAN: *Japan Publications Trading Co., Ltd., 1-2-1, Sarugaku-cho, Chiyoda-ku, Tokyo 101.*

First edition: August 1988

LCCC No. 86–62961
ISBN 0–87040–686–8

Printed in U.S.A.

Contents

Editor's Note

Edward Esko

Today, our approach to health care is changing. Leading public health agencies around the world, including the National Academy of Sciences and the National Cancer Institute, have issued dietary guidelines for the prevention of disease that parallel macrobiotics. At the same time, growing numbers of people have begun taking greater responsibility for their health, often with the encouragement of their doctors. Proper exercise, stress management, meditation, mental imaging, and other self-help techniques are a part of this trend, as is the practice of a naturally balanced diet. Meanwhile, the number of doctors, nurses, nutritionists, researchers, and other health professionals who have adopted macrobiotics is increasing. In this book you will meet doctors who represent this new type of health professional.

The principle of macrobiotics—yin and yang, or the universal law of harmony and balance—has been understood for centuries in all traditional cultures. It formed the theoretical basis for medical practice in ancient Greece and China, and was expressed in a variety of ways in the world's great religions and philosophies. This principle is especially relevant today, as it makes the cause of degenerative sickness more readily understandable, while pointing the way toward practical solutions.

A fundamental approach to preventing and recovering from disease requires an understanding of the most primary causes. Without changing the underlying factors that create sickness—especially daily diet and way of life—our approach remains symptomatic, and in many cases, carries the risk of side effects. A naturally balanced diet—one that avoids potentially harmful extremes such as the overconsumption of saturated fat, sugar, and chemicalized or irradiated foods—is an essential part of a healthful lifestyle, and fundamental to the practice of macrobiotics.

In their essays, the doctors look at health and healing from

1

this holistic perspective. They discuss the importance of a macro-biotically balanced diet in the prevention and recovery from illness, and mention the role played by factors such as family support, positive mental imaging, and stress reduction. They also present scientific data linking diet and lifestyle with cancer, heart disease, immune deficiencies, PMS, behavioral disorders, and other illnesses, and urge everyone to assume personal respon-sibility for their health and well-being. The doctors also challenge their colleagues in the medical profession to develop supportive relationships with their patients based on mutual respect and understanding.

These essays, written by men and women who have adopted macrobiotics in their lives, point to the emergence of a new model of health care based on the synthesis of East and West, traditional wisdom and modern practice, and intuitive perception and scientific analysis. This new model can lead beyond problems of personal health and toward health and harmony on a global scale.

I would like to thank everyone who participated in creating this book. I thank Michio Kushi for providing the material for the introduction, based on lectures in which he discusses the modern health crisis, including the emergence of AIDS and immune deficiencies, and introduces the macrobiotic approach. I thank all of the contributors for taking time from their busy schedules to write essays, and for their untiring dedication to human health and well-being. I also thank Lawrence H. Kushi, now at the Fred Hutchinson Cancer Research Center in Seattle, for writing the foreword, and Alex Jack, Phillip Jannetta, and members of the Japan Publications staff in Tokyo for reviewing the text and producing the finished volume.

Finally, I would like to thank Mr. Iwao Yoshizaki and Mr. Yoshiro Fujiwara, respectively president and New York re-presentative of Japan Publications, for producing this book and for their dedication to a healthy and peaceful world.

Foreword

Lawrence H. Kushi, Sc.D.

In the summer of 1985, I attended a two-week seminar on the epidemiology of cardiovascular diseases sponsored by the American Heart Association near Tahoe City, California. The opening dinner, at which seminar participants and instructors broke ice and mingled, featured good company in a beautiful setting—along with generous portions of steak. The next few days were blue-sky sunshiny days of intellectual conversation and forging of friendships, fueled by breakfasts of cholesterol-free omelets and mid-morning fruit breaks.

These few days were a study in the growing awareness of the relationship between diet and health in the biomedical community —and its as yet ambivalent acceptance. One focus of these seminars was the way in which diet affects atherosclerosis, the process that underlies most cardiovascular disease in industrialized societies. Indeed, the American Heart Association has taken a leadership role in educating the public about these relationships. Their recommendations for the prevention of heart disease suggest, among other measures, decreasing the proportion of fat in the diet to less than 30 percent of calories, and perhaps even less than 20 percent. Even so, at this meeting sponsored by this same association, the main course of the "special occasion" dinner was artery-clogging red meat. Clearly, there exists still a mind/body dissonance that results in behavior that is at odds with one's intellectual realization about the desirability of that behavior.

This meeting of the American Heart Association was a study in contrasts in other ways as well. Held at the north end of Lake Tahoe, it was just a dozen miles by hiking trail (or three and a half hours by car) from the French Meadows location of the annual macrobiotic summer camp organized by Herman and Cornellia Aihara. The mid-seminar weekend was set aside as free time, and a friend and I chose to hike over to the macrobiotic summer camp. The hike took us through the beautiful high country of the Sierra

Nevadas. We saw nary another person on the trail once we left the commercialized Squaw Valley and Lake Tahoe basin.

This overnight hike, with good food and friends at the other end of the trail, was one of the most memorable I have taken. After leaving a rustic yet lavish seminar held in a time-sharing ski resort, we hiked to a primitive National Forest campground. From a seminar with 25 participants and half as many instructors, we went to a camp with a hundred people in attendance. Both were filled with warmth and friendship. But while potential changes in behavior to prevent heart disease were discussed at the former, living examples of how this can be attained—with little or no reference to heart disease—were studying and celebrating macrobiotics at the latter.

The goals and dreams of these two groups of people are similar, but their approaches and knowledge base stand in sharp contrast with each other. The obstacles that might bring together these two approaches toward a healthful lifestyle seem as formidable as the mountains that stood between the locations of these two gatherings. Yet, just as my friend and I were able to cross the wilderness between the American Heart Association meeting and the French Meadows summer camp, so too can these two differing but complementary perspectives be joined.

The complementary nature of macrobiotics and the biomedical world is becoming increasingly clear as the nature of macrobiotics is less often misunderstood, and as the scope of medical topics continues to expand. Even in their most basic or superficial levels, however, these two clearly support each other. In macrobiotics, good food is often regarded as the basis for health. A fundamental theme of biomedical research is the increasingly clear relationship between diet and health.

In many instances, macrobiotic practice predates "official" scientific recognition of the role diet has in causing and preventing disease. For example, the East West Foundation, a non-profit organization devoted to macrobiotic education, sponsored a symposium on diet and cancer in 1974, and macrobiotic literature and teaching noted the relationship between diet and cancer well before that. In contrast, a dozen years ago, most physicians and researchers would have regarded with great skepticism the notion that diet has anything to do with the prevention or treatment of cancer. In 1982 and 1984, however, the National Academy of Sciences and the American Cancer Society published dietary recommendations for the prevention of cancer. These recommendations sounded much like actual macrobiotic dietary practice to those with an understanding of the macrobiotic way of life.

From the perspective of one living in the United States, the first "official" pronouncements regarding diet and its relationship with chronic diseases such as heart disease or cancer probably came from the American Heart Association in the early 1960's. However, the first such declaration to be widely disseminated that suggested dramatic changes in dietary habits for all people in the United States was the publication of the *U.S. Dietary Goals* in February, 1977.

There were six dietary goals outlined by the Senate Select Committee on Nutrition and Human Needs, chaired by Senator George McGovern. These goals were as follows:

1) Increase carbohydrate consumption to account for 55 to 60 percent of the energy (caloric) intake.
2) Reduce overall fat consumption from approximately 40 to 30 percent of energy intake.
3) Reduce saturated fat consumption to account for about 10 percent of total energy intake; and balance that with poly-unsaturated and monounsaturated fats, which should ac-for about 10 percent of energy intake each.
4) Reduce cholesterol consumption to about 300 mg. a day.
5) Reduce sugar consumption by about 40 percent to account count for about 15 percent of total energy intake.
6) Reduce salt consumption by about 50 to 85 percent to approximately 3 grams a day.

A subsequent revision of this publication modified two of these goals (to decrease sugar to 10 percent of total energy, and decrease salt to about 5 grams a day), and added a seventh goal of moderation of energy intake: To avoid overweight, consume only as much energy (calories) as is expended; if overweight, decrease energy intake and increase energy expenditure.

This landmark publication, which has since taken on the seemingly contradictory natures of being both prophetic and mundane, of being both quixotic and cautious, was initially criticized—not for health reasons—by those who would be hurt economically by wholesale adoption of these goals. Thus, the National Livestock and Meat Board, the Egg Board, the National Dairy Council, the Salt Institute and the International Sugar Research Foundation were all critical of these goals.

Incredibly, the American Medical Association also strongly criticized these goals. The AMA stated that "there is a potential for harmful effects from a radical long-term dietary change as would occur through adoption of the proposed national goals." Yet, it failed to provide any information to support this supposition. To some observers, it appeared that the primary motive here was also economic, to protect the livelihood of the members of this trade association (physicians), rather than to promote the health of the U.S. population. In marked contrast to the stance taken by the AMA, the respected British medical journal, the *Lancet*, stated that "The American goals will be welcomed by people who have thought seriously about the diet of modern Western man" (23 April 77).

Perhaps what was most telling about these goals was that they came not from a professional organization, such as the AMA, the American Dietetic Association or the American Society for Clinical Nutrition, nor did they come from a branch of government that dealt with the problems of diet or health, such as the Department of Agriculture, the Food and Drug Administration, or the Department of Health, Education and Welfare. Instead, these dietary goals were the work of a Senate Committee. This origin is symptomatic of a major limitation of the U.S. health care system: innovations in the area of diet and nutrition in relation to health usually occur outside professional circles before becoming well-accepted within the medical profession.

Principal examples of these innovations are the role that macro-biotics and people influenced by macrobiotics have played in changing the dietary habits of this nation. I remember the lack of availability as a young child of such basics of good nutrition as whole grains or a varied produce section in food stores. Brown rice was a gourmet specialty item, and *tofu* was a rare ethnic food found only in Japanese and Chinese restaurants.

In order to provide good quality foods to the small but growing macrobiotic community in Boston, my parents started to package in their basement different whole grains and beans for their friends and students. This eventually developed into an actual storefront operation with the opening of Erewhon in 1966, one of the first natural food stores in the country. Its decor was natural post-hippie environmentally attractive, with food available in bulk quantities and plenty of woodwork throughout. Since then, these types of stores have proliferated throughout the country. Most major cities have at least one such natural food store or cooperative, often started by an individual influenced by macrobiotics. The major natural food companies in the United States, Japan and Europe were all started by students of macrobiotics who have had the practical vision to provide good quality food to the public.

In some sense, the expansion of the natural food industry and the growing public awareness of diet and its effects on health needed to precede official recommendations regarding dietary change and health. For example, it has been said that dietary change is difficult to make because the infrastructure that would allow such change does not exist. With the availability of a wide variety of quality natural foods and foods that could be substituted for usual American-cuisine foods, real changes in diet that lower risk of chronic diseases can be achieved practically. The work of friends influenced by macrobiotics to establish a viable natural foods industry has thus been instrumental in creating a societal climate in which dietary recommendations can be made. However, this is a slowly-changing process, since many people who are in professional roles of advising dietary change are not aware of the availability of foods that come from the natural foods industry.

Since the publication of the U.S. Dietary Goals, several scientific organizations have made dietary recommendations aimed at the U.S. population. The major recommendations in this regard, aside from those of the American Heart Association, which are periodically revised as more is known of the relationship of diet with heart disease, have been: the *Surgeon General's Report on Health Promotion and Disease Prevention; Dietary Guidelines for Americans*, a joint effort of the U.S. Departments of Agriculture and Health and Human Services; *Interim Dietary Guidelines* for the prevention of cancer of the National Academy of Sciences; and, the American Cancer Society dietary recommendations for the prevention of cancer. These recommendations by and large agree with those in the U.S. Dietary Goals.

The Surgeon General's report, published in 1979, was aimed at many aspects of lifestyle, of which diet was one. The recommendations for diet stated that "People should adopt prudent dietary habits, consuming: 1) only sufficient calories to meet body needs (fewer calories if the person is overweight); 2) less saturated fat and cholesterol; 3) less salt; 4) less sugar; 5) relatively more complex carbohydrates, such as whole grains, cereals, fruits and vegetables; and 6) relatively more fish, poultry, legumes (e.g., peas, beans, peanuts), and less red meat."

Dietary Guidelines for Americans, initially published in 1980 and revised in 1981, listed the following seven recommendations: 1) eat a variety of foods; 2) maintain desirable weight; 3) avoid too much fat, saturated fat, and cholesterol; 4) eat foods with adequate starch and fiber; 5) avoid too much sugar; 6) avoid too much sodium; and, 7) if you drink alcoholic beverages, do so in moderation.

The National Academy of Science's *Interim Dietary Guidelines* for the prevention of cancer, published by its Committee on Diet, Nutrition and Cancer in 1982, were based on the conclusion that "the differences in the rates at which various cancers occur in different human populations are often correlated with differences in diet. The likelihood that some of these correlations reflect causality is strengthened by laboratory evidence that similar dietary patterns and components of food also affect the incidence of certain cancers in animals." There were six guidelines, four of which were aimed at the general population:

1) "The committee recommends that the consumption of both saturated and unsaturated fats be reduced in the average U.S. diet. An appropriate and practical target is to reduce intake from its present level (approximately 40 percent) to 30 percent of total calories in the diet. The scientific data do not provide a strong basis for establishing fat intake at precisely 30 percent of total calories. Indeed, the data could be used to justify an even greater reduction. However, in

the judgment of the committee, the suggested reduction (i.e., one-quarter of fat intake) is a moderate and practical target, and is likely to be beneficial."

2) "The committee emphasizes the importance of including fruits, vegetables, and whole grain cereal products in the daily diet."

3) "The committee recommends that the consumption of food preserved by salt-curing (including salt-pickling) or smoking be minimized."

4) "The committee recommends that if alcoholic beverages are consumed, it be done in moderation."

The other two guidelines were aimed primarily at the food industry, research organizations and regulatory agencies, and were geared toward ensuring to the extent possible that carcinogens and mutagens do not contaminate foods or are removed or minimized when naturally present in foods.

The American Cancer Society dietary recommendations for cancer prevention, published in 1984, were as follows: 1) avoid obesity; 2) cut down on total fat intake; 3) eat more high fiber foods, such as whole grain cereals, fruits and vegetables; 4) include foods rich in vitamins A and C in the daily diet; 5) include cruciferous vegetables, such as cabbage, broccoli, Brussels sprouts, kohlrabi and cauliflower in the diet; 6) be moderate in consumption of alcoholic beverages; and, 7) be moderate in consumption of salt-cured, smoked and nitrite-cured foods.

It is apparent that these dietary recommendations are quite similar to each other. In a sense, this is not surprising, since these recommendations are based on the same body of scientific literature. It is also apparent that the practical application of these recommendations are expressed in macrobiotic practice. Unlike the so-called scientific basis for the recommendations outlined above, macrobiotic dietary principles come primarily from a philosophical appreciation of the evolutionary and cultural history of humanity. Thus, the foods and dishes in macrobiotic cuisine are invariably based on traditional foods. Many of these foods have grown to be widely accepted in modern American cuisine. Examples of this include tofu and brown rice, mentioned earlier as formerly rare and now commonly available foods.

Eating macrobiotically invariably results in a diet that, compared to the typical U.S. diet, is low in fat, saturated fats, cholesterol and sugar, high in complex carbohydrates and fiber, and rich in various vitamins and minerals. This nutrient consumption pattern is a practical application of the various "official" dietary recommendations for the prevention of chronic diseases. The congruence between dietary recommendations and macrobiotic practice is somewhat less than coincidental. In 1974 and 1974, two papers that demonstrated that people eating macrobiotically had low blood pressure and low serum cholesterol levels, placing them at low risk for heart disease, were published in medical journals. These and other studies in macrobiotic and vegetarian groups are among the various sources of evidence on which these dietary recommendations are based.

The task of increasing understanding between the medical and macrobiotic communities is fundamentally the same as when strengthening relationships between any other pair and set of communities. Probably the first important step in this task is the development of personal friendships. Such ties form the basis of cooperation in working toward mutual goals such as the realization of a healthful, peaceful world. The most well-known example of the fruitfulness of such a relationship is the publication of Dr. Anthony Sattilaro's story in *Recalled by Life*. In this book, Dr. Sattilaro recounts his experience with prostatic cancer, explaining how macrobiotics helped him to recover and lead a fulfilling life. This book and his story have probably done as much to promote and increase awareness of macrobiotics as any other publication. Despite this book, and perhaps in part because of it, the American Cancer Society published a statement that denounces macrobiotics as an unproven and probably dangerous method of cancer therapy. Interestingly, this statement was published in the same journal in which they published their dietary recommendations for the prevention of cancer—and just one month apart. Clearly, there is a long way to go before it can be said that macrobiotics and the medical world have a mutually respectful relationship.

The appreciation of macrobiotics that is expressed in the various essays in this book are further examples of the understanding that can be cultivated between people in the medical community and macrobiotics. The basis of respect for macrobiotics among these physicians often springs from a personal experience of severe illness, as has been the inspiration for many other people. These people and their essays serve as examples of the first important step in development of greater acceptance and understanding of macrobiotics in the medical world: the cultivation of personal friendships among such people. There are further steps that can be taken to expand upon the friendships and communication illustrated in this book. If some of these are implemented, true cooperation between the macrobiotic and conventional medical communities may occur. Two aspects of further tasks that can be developed and pursued are outlined here.

Mutual Education

It is apparent that the primary obstacle to acceptance of macrobiotics in biomedical circles is a misconception of what macrobiotics is. Among many dietitians and physicians, macrobiotics continues to be thought of as a series of diets, one more extreme than the next. This is despite the impression I have that such an image has to a large extent disappeared among other sectors of society. Indeed, the perpetuation of misconceptions about macrobiotics may be due in part to the medical community. For example, basic nutrition textbooks continue to talk about "food faddism," with the macrobiotic diet usually given as an example of the most extreme of such diets. In part, this view is justified because of the inappropriate practice of macrobiotics that has led to case histories of individuals who have developed scurvy (vitamin C deficiency, brought about by the exclusive consumption of grains), or vitamin B_{12} deficiency. The simple illustration that this image of macrobiotics is incorrect would go a long way toward placing the macrobiotic lifestyle in a more favorable light. Indeed, such has been my experience when talking with other researchers about the general practice and understanding of macrobiotics. When the brown-rice only misconception of macrobiotics is put to rest, macrobiotics is suddenly cast in the light of being a healthy approach to eating, but one that is perhaps impractical for most Americans. The arena of debate about macrobiotics is then no longer in the realm of "the craziness of that diet," but is instead in the area of discussing the practicalities and potential health benefits of eating macrobiotically.

Misconceptions about modern medicine abound in macrobiotic circles as well. Too often, the medical community is thought of as a technological, unfeeling, impersonal monstrosity that fosters and perpetuates illness rather than promotes health. Indeed, there is justification for such a view, just as there is a basis for the idea that macrobiotics is an extreme diet that causes malnutrition. For example, hospitals often measure success in terms of how many operations they have carried out, rather than priding themselves for the number of seemingly necessary operations they were able to avoid. Physicians are often quick to embrace new medications to lower cholesterol levels even though it has been demonstrated that a concerted dietary change can be far more effective with many fewer side effects. The reaction of the macrobiotic community to such obviously misplaced priorities is too often the rejection of all things medical. Paradoxically, an equally strong reaction is the reverence toward physicians who show an appreciation for macrobiotics. Both reactions may be tempered and humanized by an understanding that the medical community is made up of people, just like other human communities.

The middle ground that enhances communication is the education of both physicians and macrobiotic practitioners in the nuances of each other's perspectives. Formal examples of this include the evolving curriculum of the Kushi Institute which attempts to explore various views of diet and nutrition, including conventional views; and the development of a physicians' education program in macrobiotics, organized by the Kushi Foundation with the cooperation of medical doctors. Further pursuit of these and similar ideas will enhance the mutual respect that can exist on an individual level, and which would provide a context for further understanding and cooperation.

Continued and Further Research

The few biomedical research studies that have examined people following a macrobiotic lifestyle have played an integral role in the growing acceptance of macrobiotics, in both the medical community and in society at large. Such studies have demonstrated that people consuming a macrobiotic diet are at dramatically lower risk for heart disease, and at possible lower risk of breast cancer. These studies have also shown that a narrow interpretation of macrobiotic dietary practice may lead to undue risk of vitamin B_{12} and vitamin D deficiency in infants. Information provided by such studies can lead to better understanding of macrobiotics, for both proponents and critics of macrobiotics.

A current example of research that has enhanced the credibility of macrobiotics is the ongoing survey of men in New York City with Acquired Immunodeficiency Syndrome who have chosen to follow a macrobiotic lifestyle. Although the number of men has been small and the study is not a "controlled" study, the attempt to obtain objective data regarding the efficacy of macrobiotics is a worthwhile effort. The experience of these men has demonstrated that at the very least, macrobiotic practice has not further harmed them, and that perhaps some indication of benefit exists. Despite the equivocal nature of these results, they have been of enough interest to encourage the government of the People's Republic of the Congo to pursue further studies on the possible benefit of macrobiotics for AIDS.

There are further areas in which research will enhance understanding of macrobiotics, and will promote communication and cooperation between the macrobiotic and medical communities. Two major areas involve the study of the efficacy of a macrobiotic diet in the treatment of diseases. One stumbling block in the credibility of macrobiotics has been the generally unsubstantiated claims made about the ability of macrobiotics to effect recovery from diseases such as lung or pancreatic cancer, which for all intents and purposes can be regarded as incurable by conventional medical therapies. Indeed, much has been made of various case histories of individuals who have conquered one disease or another by following macrobiotic recommendations. Dr. Sattilaro's story is the most well-known example of this.

Despite the claims of macrobiotic proponents, it has often been pointed out that such case histories are the weakest of sources of evidence of the benefits of macrobiotics. The most convincing demonstration of the benefit of macrobiotics would come only from a randomized clinical trial of its effects on one disease or another. In theory, such studies are possible, but they would require more resources than most funding sources would be willing to make available. This unwillingness is based primarily on the paucity of objective studies that have looked at macrobiotics—or any aspect of diet—in the treatment of cancer or other diseases.

In order to enhance the possibility of conducting such studies, the first step would probably be the systematization of records kept by those who provide education to people with severe illnesses who seek information about macrobiotics. The next needed component may be the regular follow-up of these individuals to determine how well they follow the recommendations, and to monitor how their health status progresses. These procedures would lead to a growing registry from which accurate statements about the effects of macrobiotic practice can be made. Information would thus be available not only on those individuals who are willing to speak out about their success with macrobiotics, but also on the others who may not have followed macrobiotics well, or who may have done poorly with macrobiotics. Such information could theoretically provide justification for the pursuit of more rigorous studies into the efficacy of macrobiotics.

An additional area in which research into macrobiotics can provide useful information is through the long-term follow-up of people following a macrobiotic lifestyle. On the occasions when a well-known person within the macrobiotic community develops an illness such as cancer, it has been remarked that "s/he couldn't have been practicing macrobiotics." Such a statement assumes, incorrectly, that macrobiotics will prevent all such diseases. What is likely true is that the risk of developing such diseases is much less among those practicing macrobiotics. However, this is based on supposition rather than actual observation, since no such study has ever been conducted. This is partly because modern-day macrobiotics is a recent phenomenon, and thus there have not been many people who would call themselves macrobiotic who have lived long enough to develop a disease such as cancer. It is also partly because it is difficult, if not impossible, to determine who is macrobiotic. Yet, such study and observation would be useful for the understanding of the long-term health benefits of macrobiotics.

A long-term study of people who follow a macrobiotic lifestyle would also require a substantial amount of money, especially if such a study were to include the collection of blood samples or conducting clinical tests such as for blood pressure. However, if such a study were conducted primarily through mail question-naires, large numbers of people could be followed for several years. In fact, such a study is currently being planned, in which not only people practicing macrobiotics, but other people follow-ing other dietary habits will be followed. Such an approach will then allow comparison of the experience of those eating macro-biotically with those who follow other dietary habits.

There are numerous other examples of studies that would en-hance the credibility of macrobiotics, while also contributing to knowledge about the general health and condition of all people. Participation by individuals in such studies may require some time and a slight feeling of "guinea pig-itis". Yet, the potential benefit to humanity of objectifying the claims of macrobiotic proponents can be enormous if there is any truth to these claims. Virtually every indication of macrobiotic experience and research in diet and health suggests that such claims have some truth to them. Investigation of such claims through the tools provided by research methodology would provide a common knowledge base that would enhance further understanding and acceptance of macrobiotics.

During the return hike from the French Meadows macrobiotic summer camp to the American Heart Association seminar near Tahoe City, I was again alone on the hiking trail. Again, the day was beautiful, and the hike peaceful and relaxing. The rustling of leaves on a summer breeze and the rhythms of my body were the only sounds to accompany me on the trail. Twice, I noticed —and was noticed by—deer as they bound alongside the trail, stopping momentarily to gaze at this human intruder in their environment before starting again on their way. At such times, the insignificance of individual human activity becomes apparent, and the joy of living with nature overwhelms other thoughts. At such times, one easily questions the purpose behind our fascination with the medical profession, or with the benefits of macro-biotics, or with the pursuit of "objective" justification for living according to the order of the universe. Could we not enjoy life as simply and effortlessly as the deer appear to?

A return to the American Heart Association seminar leads to the realization that the answers to such queries are not so easy. The need for large changes in society are apparent, in the continuing toll that cancer and cardiovascular diseases have in our society. The fact that such diseases are largely preventable, yet even the leaders of American society regarding knowledge of prevention are reluctant to act on that knowledge underlines the extent to which macrobiotics can contribute to the betterment of society. With the respected role that physicians and the scientific method hold in our society, the development of understanding and research into the effects of macrobiotics are vital.

Even the pursuit of such understanding is only a stepping stone toward reversing other trends in society. The link between personal dietary consciousness and concern for global well-being is direct and interdependent. This link is fed directly by a marriage of the respect for nature that is a fundamental aspect of macrobiotics with the open yet skeptical search for understanding that is basic to scientific inquiry. Indeed, the beauty of a deer as it leaps over fallen timber is compelling reason for bringing the compassion and respect for nature that is a fundamental aspect of macrobiotics to the analytic approach of conventional medicine. The joint contributions of the philosophical and scientific, of the heart and the mind will be necessary to achieve a peaceful world society. The bridging of gaps as shown in the accompanying essays are the first small steps toward these goals.

Introduction

Michio Kushi

More than twenty years ago, I met with a group of doctors at a New York hospital to discuss macrobiotics. I stated that America and the rest of the modern world would end if we did not change our way of thinking, lifestyle, and way of eating. I used the increase in cancer as an example of the degenerative trends that threatened modern society.

The doctors shrugged their shoulders and glanced at each other with puzzled expressions. They could not understand what I was saying, and several actively disagreed. At that time, research was concentrating on the virus theory, the hereditary theory, and a variety of other theories about the cause of cancer. There was little awareness of the environmental causes of cancer, including the relationship between diet and cancer.

Five years later, I met with a group of professors at Harvard and presented the same idea. Several answered, "Well possibly," while the others did not actively oppose what I had said. Perhaps they were only being polite.

Nearly five years later, I met with President Carter's advisors in Washington, D. C. A handful of advisors were present at this meeting where I offered the same view. I recommended that the United States change its agricultural, food, and health policies in order to avert future catastrophe. Several of the advisors shook their heads as if they did not understand or disagreed. But to my surprise, the majority nodded in agreement.

Now, people are becoming more aware of the situation and are starting to worry about the rising tide of biological degeneration. A brief look at statistics gathered from medical and public health sources can help us understand the scope of the problem.

Out of a population of about 230 million, about 43 million people in the United States currently suffer from heart and cardiovascular disease, nearly 20 percent of the entire population. About 37 million have high blood pressure; and 36 million suffer from allergies. About 32 million—or roughly 15 percent of the population—suffer from arthritis. About 11 million have diabetes, and there are about 1.8 million strokes every year in this country. Currently, one out of three people in the United States is expected to develop cancer at some point in their lives. Forty years ago, the rate was about one out of seven.

About 25 percent of the American population will suffer at some time from some form of mental illness, and about 10 percent require care. A large number of these people will become disabled because of mental illness; they will be unable to work or function normally.

Reproductive abilities have declined in the twentieth century. Infertility affects about one out of five American couples. According to one study, average sperm counts in Western men have dropped approximately 30 percent over the last sixty years, and it is estimated that as many as 20 percent of young men do not have the ability to fertilize an ovum. Their sperm counts are either too low, their sperm are too weak, or they are sexually incapable.

Every year, about 700,000 to 800,000 American women undergo hysterectomies, so that by the age of sixty-five, 50 percent have no ovaries or uterus. In the last few years, herpes and other sexually transmitted diseases (STD) have assumed epidemic proportions. Conservative estimates are that 20 to 30 million Americans are now infected with the herpes virus, for which there is no medical cure.

In the 1980s, a new disease emerged from nowhere to capture public attention and concern. This condition, *Acquired Immune Deficiency Syndrome*, or *AIDS*, could become the world's leading health problem during the remainder of this century and into the next.

At the present time, as many as three million people in the United States could be harboring the AIDS virus. According to estimates based on recent experience, the number of people with the virus doubles every year. If the virus spreads this rapidly, it is theoretically possible that by 1994, the number of people carrying it could exceed the U.S. population.

Of the people carrying the virus, as many as one-third could go on to develop acute AIDS, and another one-third *AIDS Related Complex* (ARC) or associated conditions. In a worst-case scenario, millions of people in the United States and other modern nations could develop the disease, and these countries could experience widespread economic and social chaos as a result. Currently, the cost of treating AIDS medically averages about $120,000 per case. If we multiply this by the potential number of cases over the next fifteen to twenty years, we see how staggering the direct medical costs of AIDS could become.

What is the extent of modern knowledge about these degenerative conditions? Practically speaking, we know very little about what causes them or how to prevent them. As a result, we are unable to make these figures decline.

Recently, people have started to realize that heart disease is caused by what we eat: foods such as beef, pork, and others that are high in saturated fat and cholesterol. Many people in the United States have reduced their meat consumption, and as a result, the rates of heart disease have started to decline. But the incidence of other degenerative diseases, including cancer and AIDS, show no signs of decreasing.

One hundred years ago, cancer research began at Sloan Kettering in New York. At that time, the cancer rate was small, similar to the present rate of AIDS. A century later, we know almost as little about the causes of the disease as we did then. AIDS presents us with another dilemma. The disease is thought to be caused by a virus, but there is still no precise understanding of the way in which the virus is transmitted, or how it interacts with the various cofactors that weaken natural immunity.

Even if the virus spreads only half as rapidly as described above, within ten years, a majority of adults in the United States could be harboring it. When the virus was first discovered, some researchers were hoping that a vaccine would be found within five years. Some even thought that compulsory vaccination of the entire population, including children, would halt the spread of the disease. However, by the time a vaccine is found—if one is ever found—tens of millions of people in the United States could already be carrying the virus, and it would not help them. As everyone knows, there is no cure for AIDS. On average, people with acute cases die within 29 months after being diagnosed. About 60 percent die within two years, and practically all die within five years.

We can summarize the problems with an AIDS vaccine in the following points:

1. As mentioned above, even if a vaccine is discovered in five years, it will not help those people already carrying the virus, including those with active cases of AIDS; and
2. No one knows what side effects an AIDS vaccine could produce. A new, more serious disease could arise as a result of exposure; the vaccine could cause the virus to mutate and become stronger, producing an even more horrible condition.

Initial optimism about finding a vaccine faded after it was discovered that the virus changes very rapidly. It is even possible that the virus differs slightly from person to person, or changes according to each person's daily condition and activity. The changeability of the virus has caused increasing confusion among researchers.

Three major health problems—cancer, AIDS, and mental illness—are at the heart of the modern crisis. Together they could cause the end of America and the rest of the modern civilized world. This end, in which people will not be able to maintain modern civilized systems, could come very soon.

Meanwhile, life goes on as usual. People are walking on the street, shopping malls are filled with customers, trains and buses are running, and rush-hour traffic is congested. As a result, most of us are too preoccupied to realize how serious the situation is.

Only a decade ago, few people paid attention to the problem of cancer. For many, cancer was remote. But now it is a problem for every family. Today, AIDS seems remote to many people; a common impression is that it occurs mostly in places like New York or San Francisco, or that it affects a minority of people in the so-called high-risk groups. But in a short time, AIDS could become everyone's problem. Every family may have to deal with it, just as they are now doing with cancer. And just as modern medicine has failed to prevent the spread of cancer and other degenerative diseases, a fundamental way of preventing AIDS is also unlikely. Even if symptomatic treatments for acute AIDS are discovered, they would not stop the constant spread of the disease. Moreover, symptomatic treatments for AIDS could cause serious side effects, just as chemotherapy, radiotherapy, and similar treatments often do in many cases.

In the Middle Ages, a plague known as the "Black Death" ravaged Europe. Millions of Europeans—almost a third of the population—perished. But AIDS and other modern degenerative diseases have a far greater potential for human destruction.

Compared to this crisis, environmental or economic issues, such as clean water or the ups and downs of the stock market, are small. The number-one issue today is whether or not humanity will survive on this planet. Of course pollution, nuclear waste, and other environmental issues are related to this crisis, and are making survival more difficult, but the key issue is each person's health and biological integrity.

Fortunately, a growing number of people, including those in the medical and scientific fields, have become aware of this crisis, and are seeking holistic and natural solutions. I appreciate their efforts very much, including past and present research on the application of macrobiotics for human health and well-being. Our macrobiotic associates, including the doctors who wrote essays for this book, are seeking the key to prevent and recover from degenerative conditions so that humanity may survive and develop toward an unlimited future.

My first encounter with AIDS occurred more than five years ago when several people with the condition came to Boston for macrobiotic advice. At that time, AIDS was not as widespread as it is today. As a result of meeting them, I became very interested in this problem. As I studied it in depth, I discovered its potential to destroy modern civilization, and began to see a relationship between immune deficiencies and the modern diet and way of life.

Shortly afterward, I, my wife, Aveline, and senior macrobiotic teachers such as Edward Esko went to New York to speak about

AIDS and macrobiotics. As I became more involved, I realized that without a facility where AIDS patients could stay, study, and eat well-prepared meals, it would be difficult to help them.

Aveline, my son, Lawrence Kushi, who at that time was doing nutritional research at the University of Minnesota, and other friends began to look for a residential facility in New England. When they contacted hospitals, they were told by the administration that macrobiotic programs would be welcome. One hospital even offered to install a gas range for cooking. But once it was stated that the program was for AIDS patients, they quickly changed their minds. One administrator said, "If your project was for cancer, diabetes, or heart disease, we would be happy to provide a facility. But not for AIDS."

We then contacted religious organizations. Like the hospitals, they were interested in making facilities available for macrobiotic programs. However, as soon as we mentioned AIDS, they all withdrew. One representative told us, "Personally I don't mind, but if the board of directors found out, they would oppose the project. If people discovered that AIDS patients were here, they would stop coming."

Faced with these responses, we decided that for the time being, the best way to help people with AIDS would be to begin regular educational programs in New York. *Wipe Out AIDS* was a local organization set up to help people with the disease. Lectures were arranged and I started to go every two months. Aveline also gave cooking classes. Several hundred people would gather at public schools and community centers in Greenwich Village for each event.

In the beginning, I was uncertain about the best way to present macrobiotics to people with AIDS. Practically every person with the disease was fearful, depressed, and desperate. Wherever they looked, they were told there was no hope. They were like plants that had withered. Their future seemed dark.

To inspire them with hope, I had to talk more happily. I even sang songs during the lectures. After several visits, more and more people with AIDS started to eat macrobiotically. Once, in the middle of a cooking class, a young man broke down and cried. "This is our only hope," he said.

Macrobiotics attempts to restore immune abilities through the most natural methods. A decline in natural immunity means there is a problem with the blood, especially the white blood cells. In order to strengthen the blood and restore immunity, people with AIDS must drastically change what they eat.

So as to better understand natural immunity, we need to consider it in light of the traditional understanding of yin and yang, which forms the basis of macrobiotic practice.

Understanding and applying yin and yang—the two primary energies in nature—is essential if we wish to achieve harmony with our changing environment. Yin and yang represent the primary forces of expansion, or centrifugal force or motion, and contraction, or centripetal force or motion found throughout nature. Both exist in everything.

For example, in the world of energy that extends beyond the senses, yin and yang exist in the form of short and long wave, and high and low frequency vibrations. Among the preatomic particles created from the condensation of energy, more yang, positively charged protons are counterbalanced by more yin, negatively charged electrons. The spirallic structure of the atom—maintained by the forces of yin and yang—is duplicated in the solar system: comets and planets orbit around a central nucleus, the sun.

The world of elements arises from the interaction of preatomic particles, and here we find lighter, more yin elements with simpler atomic structures, and heavier, more yang elements with complex atomic structures.

Elements also pass constantly through stages from the more yin, diffused stages of plasma, gas, and liquid, to the more yang, compact or solid stage.

Earth's climatic regions also balance yin and yang. More cold, northern climates counterbalance warmer equatorial regions. Dry regions, which are more yang, exist in counterpoint to more yin, humid regions, and more yin higher altitudes contrast with more yang plains and valleys. To balance these natural environments, living things—plants and animals—become more yang or compacted as the surroundings become colder, and become more expanded and yin as the environment becomes hotter.

Yin and yang also exist in the realm of biological life. Plants counterbalance animals. More yin, cold-blooded, water-dwelling, and primitive species of animal life contrast with more yang, warm-blooded, land-dwelling, and more highly evolved species.

All of the structures and functions of the human body can also be understood in terms of yin and yang. Internal organs, for example, function in complementary pairs, with more yang, compact organs making balance with more yin, structurally expanded organs. The compact heart is counterbalanced by the more expanded small intestine, the lungs by the large intestine, the liver by the gall bladder, the spleen and pancreas by the stomach, and the kidneys by the bladder.

Within the endocrine system, more yang hormones, such as insulin, testosterone, and *oxytocin* (which stimulates birth contractions) are counterbalanced by more yin hormones such as anti-insulin, estrogen, and *prolactin* (which stimulates lactation).

Complementary distinctions exist in the nervous system between the more yin peripheral nervous system and the more yang central nervous system, and between the parasympathetic and ortho-sympathetic branches of the autonomic nervous system.

The flow of blood throughout the body is counterbalanced by the flow of lymph fluid, and within the bloodstream, more yang red blood cells are counterbalanced by more yin white blood cells, or *lymphocytes.*

Yin and yang also help clarify the relationship between food, environment, and health and sickness. Health represents a dynamic condition of balance between the human body and the environment. Daily food and drink are the intermediaries between the two, and are the key to maintaining balance and harmony, or to developing imbalance and disharmony.

General Yin (▽) and Yang (△) Classification of Food

Strong Yang Foods: *
Refined salt
Eggs
Meat
Hard cheese

Chicken and poultry
Fish (especially red-meat and blue-skinned varieties)
Seafood

More Balanced Foods:
Whole cereal grains
Beans and bean products
Root, round, and leafy green vegetables (from temperate zones)
Sea vegetables
Unrefined sea salt, vegetable oil, and other natural seasonings
  (when used moderately)
Spring or well water
Non-aromatic, non-stimulant teas and beverages
Seeds and nuts
Temperate-climate fruit
Rice syrup, barley malt, and other natural-grain-based sweeteners
(when used moderately)

Strong Yin Foods:
White rice, white flour
Frozen and canned foods
Tropical fruits and vegetables (including those originating in the
  tropics such as tomato and potato)
Milk, cream, yogurt, and ice cream
Refined oils
Spices (pepper, curry, nutmeg, etc.)
Aromatic and stimulant beverages (coffee, black tea, mint tea, etc.)
Honey, sugar, and refined sweeteners
Alcohol

---

* Note that in the strong yang column, items are listed from most contractive (refined salt and eggs) to least contractive (fish and seafood), which
are thus more suitable for occasional consumption if desired. In the
strong yin column, items are listed from least expansive (white rice and
white flour) to most expansive (drugs and many medications). Foods in
the center column are generally listed from those of most central balance
(whole cereal grains, beans, vegetables, and sea vegetables) that are recommended for daily consumption to those of lesser balance (fruits and
natural sweeteners) that are recommended for occasional consumption in
moderate volume.

Foods containing chemicals, preservatives, dyes, pesticides
Drugs (marijuana, cocaine, etc., with some exceptions)
Medications (tranquilizers, antibiotics, etc., with some exceptions)

An example of the way that yin and yang work in the human body can be found in the common practice of using aspirin to prevent heart attack and stroke.

Aspirin is an extreme yin, or expansive substance. It can cause side effects such as upset stomach, nausea, vomiting, and in high doses, bleeding in the stomach or intestines. Despite its side effects, however, close to 80 million aspirin tablets are consumed every day in the United States. Aspirin also has an anti-clotting effect: one tablet can delay the time it takes for a small wound to heal, from an average of about three minutes to six. When combined with another more yin substance—alcohol—it can prolong bleeding for more than 20 minutes or cause hemorrhaging. Aspirin also reduces the rate at which hard fats accumulate in the blood vessels, and that is why some people take it in hopes of lowering their risk of heart disease.

As we discuss in the book, *Diet for a Strong Heart* (St. Martin's Press, 1985), there are two broad categories of cardiovascular disease. In one, deposits of saturated fat and cholesterol accumulate in the blood vessels, and sometimes lead to the formation of blood clots. These accumulations, and the narrowing of the blood vessels that can result, are accelerated by overconsumption of more extreme yang, or contractive foods, including eggs, meat, hard cheese, and refined salt. A stroke that occurs when a clot interferes with the flow of blood to the brain is an example of this type of disorder. Aspirin, which has an opposite, or more yin effect, can sometimes offset these symptoms.

However, the other category of cardiovascular disorder results from an opposite cause: overintake of extreme yin, or expansive foods and beverages, including alcohol, sugar, soft drinks, and tropical fruits. These items expand blood volume and increase outward pressure on the blood vessels. In extreme cases, the blood vessels in the brain erupt, and the resulting hemorrhage also produces a stroke. According to the Harvard Stroke Registry, about 16 percent of the strokes in this country are of this type, and are opposite in nature to those mentioned above. Rather than helping these conditions, aspirin, which is also yin, can cause them to become worse. As one stroke specialist recently told the *Boston Globe*, "Aspirin is no good for hemorrhage."

Health is the result of a proper balance of yin and yang factors in our daily diet and way of life. When the balance between these factors becomes extreme or one-sided, sickness is the natural result. Let us now consider the problem of AIDS and immune deficiencies from the point of view of yin and yang.*

Cold, northern places like Canada or the Soviet Union normally have fewer cases of AIDS than southern, warmer areas like Brazil or central Africa. AIDS is also more prevalent among homosexuals than it is among heterosexuals. These are indications that AIDS is a more yin condition.

Practically all of the people I have met with AIDS used marijuana, cocaine, heroin, and other drugs, all of which are extremely yin. Other yin extremes, including the overintake of fats, such as those in dairy products, and simple sugars like those in refined sugar, chocolate, carob, honey, and tropical fruits can also weaken immune response.

T-cells and *B-cells* are among the varieties of white blood cells, or lymphocytes, that are responsible for sustaining natural immunity. Among T-cells, some are more yin and others are more yang.

If a foreign substance enters the body, for example, a more yin type of virus, the more yang variety of T-cell immediately reacts and signals the B-cells. The B-cells respond according to the type of signal they receive. If the signals originate from more yang T-cells, the B-cells secrete a more yang substance, or antibody, that complements the virus. The antibody and virus immediately attract and cancel each other out.

Immune response is simply a process of harmony between yin and yang. If a more yang type of virus enters the body, more yin T-cells act and signal the B-cells to produce more yin antibodies.

---

* For a more complete presentation of the macrobiotic view of AIDS, please see *AIDS*: *Cause and Solution—The Macrobiotic Approach to Natural Immunity*, by Michio Kushi and Martha Cottrell, M.D., Japan Publications, 1988

Since contagious viruses are usually more yin, the first process —in which more yang antibodies are produced—occurs most often. If this process does not work, it is because the T-cells —especially more yang T-cells—and the B-cells have become weak and cannot respond adequately.

In attempting to confront the virus, modern approaches sidestep the issue of weakened immunity. The virus is considered the enemy, and efforts are focused on blocking or destroying it, while the immune system is often described as a battlefield. The virus is a "foreign invader." The T-cells are the body's "early warning system"; the B-cells, the body's "defense command centers" that launch "missiles," or antibodies, that "seek out and destroy the enemy." But in the macrobiotic view, a virus activates the T-cells which signal the B-cells to produce substances that complement it. In other words, the immune response is a process of natural harmony, not war.

Modern researchers are constantly searching for new weapons in a never-ending battle against disease. And, in the case of immune deficiencies, the importance of strengthening the T-cells, B-cells, or functioning of the body as a whole is overlooked.

What is the most fundamental way to restore natural immunity? Our blood, including the immune cells, is made from what we eat and drink. So by changing our food, we change the plasma, or liquid portion of the blood, as well as the red blood cells and lymphocytes, including T- and B-cells. By avoiding the excessive dietary factors that weaken immunity, and eating in accord with the natural order, the body can begin producing healthy immune cells, and the natural process of harmonization, which is the immune response, can again begin to function.

In general, someone with AIDS must gradually become more yang in order to restore natural immunity. However, if they take plenty of strong yang food, for example salt, they will begin to crave strong yin, such as sugar or tropical fruit, and thus make their condition worse. The intake of strong yang can also cause excessive factors stored in the body to discharge more actively. An overly yang diet could cause a discharge symptom such as *Kaposi's sarcoma*, the type of skin cancer that many people with

AIDS have, to proliferate. Therefore, we cannot simply think that because AIDS is more yin, people with this condition should eat more yang. The key is to provide a natural diet that properly balances both energies.

Weapons are unnecessary with this approach. However, in order to find the best weapons against cancer, AIDS, and other illnesses, 70 million animals are killed for research purposes in the United States every year. Our modern health-care system is based on destruction and sacrifice.

As long as we hold to a destructive or defensive view of the world, solutions to the problem of health and sickness will remain elusive. We will be unable to discover the peaceful, natural process of harmony that occurs in the human body and throughout nature. There is no war taking place in our body or in the universe. Sickness is not our enemy. The modern notion of "cell wars" is based on an imaginary view of the human body as a battleground, and is not reality at all.

The universe exists as a beautiful order. Everything is moving and changing according to that order, including health and sickness, emotions and feelings, and the movement of society. The order of the universe is the order of harmony, in which there are no destructive factors. We see the universe as violent because of an unhealthy brain quality.

These illusions naturally give rise to fear. Because of fear, we either attack first and try to destroy whatever we think is the enemy, or we mobilize for defense. Modern defense industries, as well as medical, insurance, police, and legal systems, are all based on the notion that life is a constant battle or struggle.

As long as we have this view, we can never find peace or happiness. We are faced with never-ending war and struggle, and cannot see how wonderful this universe is. We live in a hell of our own making.

As our educational programs continued in New York, researchers from the Boston University School of Medicine began monitoring the progress of the men who were practicing macrobiotics. The research included recording immune parameters such as total lymphocyte and T4 cell counts. In a July, 1985 letter to the British medical journal, *Lancet*, entitled, "Patients with Kaposi's Sarcoma Who Opt for No Treatment," the researchers reported on the study:

"At the International AIDS Conference in Atlanta last April someone asked if it would be ethical to include a control or placebo group in drug trials in Kaposi's sarcoma (KS). The implication was that the lack of treatment would reduce survival. This does not seem to be so. Since May, 1984, we have been studying immune function in a group which includes ten men with KS who have chosen not to enter conventional treatment protocols. Eight are still alive an average of 21.5 months after diagnosis (range 13–37 months). One person died 11 and another 20 months after diagnosis. Two of the men had opportunistic infections (OI) 18 and 21 months after diagnosis. Three of the men have had localized radiation therapy for their KS five, 18 (one of the men who had an OI and died), and 29 months after diagnosis. The others have not received medical treatment for their KS, nor have they been inpatients since the diagnosis. Most are still working.

"These men seem to be surviving at least as well as patients who have been treated. The average survival rate for men with KS alone in New York is 29 months. The average survival for men with KS and Pneumocystis carinii pneumonia or other OI is about 14 months.

"These men in our study may not be representative of KS patients in general. Their choice to forgo conventional medical therapy may indicate a strong, independent psychological make-up which could enhance survival. They are all following a vegetarian (macrobiotic) diet and have a strong social support system. They at first had minimal disease with KS lesions diagnosed only on the skin and palate. Their T4/T8 ratio, which reportedly correlates with survival, is higher than that reported for patients with KS (0.7=0.4, n=8 vs. 0.4=0.3, n=95) (mean =SD).

"Survival in these men who have received little or no medical treatment appears to compare very favorably with that of KS patients in general. We suggest that physicians and scientists can feel comfortable in allowing patients, particularly those with minimal disease, to go untreated as part of a larger study or because non-treatment is the patient's choice.

"Several drugs are being evaluated or will soon be evaluated in clinical trials. These trials should be scientific and include a placebo control group. The survival of men with KS for longer than three years with no medical intervention indicates that occasional "successes" in uncontrolled treatment protocols may in fact reflect part of the spectrum of the natural course of the disease that is favored by as yet undefined host and/or extrinsic factors rather than an effect of a particular drug."

In a January 1986 letter, Elinor Levy and John Beldekas of the Department of Microbiology at Boston University commented on the macrobiotic-AIDS research:

"The results of our ongoing study of men with AIDS who are macrobiotic are encouraging. We have been studying men sequentially since May 1984 to follow certain immune parameters. At present the data suggest a stabilization of the % T4 positive cells and lymphocyte number in about 50% of the group. The general pattern in people with KS is a steady decline in both % T4 and total lymphocyte number. This is thought to be a significant indicator of morbidity. Therefore, the ability to stabilize these parameters, in so large a proportion of our study group, is a hopeful sign."

The first step in restoring natural immunity is to improve the overall quality of the blood, including the cells of the immune system, through a balanced natural diet. Several years ago, researchers at Harvard Medical School and Ghent University in Belgium studied the blood of people who were eating macrobiotically. They were astonished at the results. First, all nutrient factors were well balanced. Secondly, the blood samples were all very clean. Third, the amount of blood fats, including cholesterol, were all very low.

Before they studied the macrobiotic blood, the researchers had thought that ideal cholesterol levels ranged between 150 to 170 mg/dl. In this range, there is little risk of arteriosclerosis or heart attack. But after they studied the blood samples of more than 200 people eating macrobiotically, their view began to change. The samples were taken by the Harvard researchers and sent to the Framingham Heart Study, one of the original epidemiological studies of heart disease, for analysis. The cholesterol levels were so low that the people at Framingham thought that the blood must have been diluted. So they called Harvard and asked, "Did you do something to this blood?" The Harvard researchers replied, "No, we just took the samples and sent them directly to you."

All of the macrobiotic people had cholesterol levels that were below 170 mg/dl. The overwhelming majority were below 150. Several were below 100, for example, 80 and 90. These are the levels of cholesterol found in children. The researchers also checked the blood pressures of more than 200 macrobiotic people and found them to be ideal; much lower than the normally high averages in the United States.

Commenting on the macrobiotic cholesterol levels, Dr. William Castelli, director of the Framingham Heart Study said, "These are levels at which we rarely, if ever, see heart disease."

Later, the Harvard team presented these results at a gathering of scientists. Another group of researchers had reported earlier on a study of people living in the South Pacific. The Pacific islanders had below average blood pressures, very low cholesterol, and no incidence of heart attack. The authors of the study felt that these favorable levels were environmentally caused: the people were living in clean, natural surroundings with none of the stresses of modern life.

Then the Harvard team reported that the macrobiotic people were maintaining almost exactly the same type of blood while living in the middle of civilization, in Boston, a stressful modern city. They stated that these results were not due to a lack of stress but to diet.

From then on, the view of heart disease underwent a change. Nutritionists and public health agencies started to actively recommend eating whole grains and vegetables as a way of preventing heart disease, even though they did not use the word "macrobiotics." The Harvard studies also influenced *Dietary*

Goals for the United States, published in 1977 by the Senate Select Committee on Nutrition and Human Needs.

Similar studies were done in Ghent, Belgium, on macrobiotic people there. The researchers found similar results, and began themselves to eat macrobiotically. I met with them later, and they told me they were planning further research, especially a controlled study to see if the macrobiotic diet could reverse arteriosclerosis.

When compared to people who eat the modern diet, the macrobiotic cholesterol levels were predictably lower. But even when compared to so-called vegetarian diets, including lacto-vegetarian and others, macrobiotic people were found to have the most favorable blood levels.

General dietary and way of life guidelines for strengthening natural immunity are presented below. Many of the recommendations parallel those presented by the National Academy of Sciences in their 1982 report, *Diet, Nutrition, and Cancer*; the Senate Select Committee on Nutrition and Human Needs, in their 1977 report, *Dietary Goals for the United States*; and preventive dietary guidelines issued by other public health agencies throughout the world. A more complete explanation of the standard macrobiotic diet is presented in the appendix, and in other books listed in the bibliography. (A summary of the research linking diet with cancer, heart disease, and other illnesses is presented in the *Book of Macrobiotics*, revised edition, by Michio Kushi with Alex Jack, Japan Publications, 1986.)

Dietary Recommendations

1. Increase the consumption of complex carbohydrates and reduce simple sugars.
2. Increase the intake of high-fiber foods and reduce those with no fiber.
3. Emphasize the use of unsaturated fat and decrease saturated fats.
4. Change from refined salt to more traditionally processed sea salt which contains trace minerals.
5. Emphasize more natural vitamins and minerals, those con-

tained within foods, and reduce intake of artificial vitamins and enzymes in supplemental form, unless it is required temporarily.

6. Increase the consumption of more natural, organically cultivated food and reduce heavily chemicalized foods.
7. Increase the intake of whole unrefined foods and reduce heavily artificialized foods.
8. Increase the use of vegetable-quality protein and reduce animal-quality protein.
9. Shift to more nutritionally balanced food from unbalanced food.
10. Shift to more economically affordable food from uneconomical and expensive foods.
11. Shift to energy saving foods from foods requiring a larger investment of energy (comparing the energy output from foods).
12. Shift to more naturally processed foods from foods that are artificially produced for commercial purposes.
13. Select food that is prepared and cooked using more traditional methods rather than fast food prepared for quick turnover.

Daily Application

1. Approximately 50 percent of the volume of food consumed daily can be whole cereal grains such as brown rice, barley, millet, whole wheat, whole oats, corn, buckwheat, rye, and whole grain products, including sourdough bread, pasta, whole wheat noodles, and others.
2. Approximately 5 to 10 percent of the volume of food consumed daily can be soup consisting of a variety of vegetables, sea vegetables, grains, beans, and occasionally fish.
3. Approximately 20 to 30 percent of the volume of food consumed daily can be vegetables prepared using various cooking styles, such as steaming, boiling, sautéing, frying, pickling, and occasionally, raw salad.
4. Approximately 5 to 10 percent of the volume of daily food

consumed can be beans of various kinds and bean products, as well as sea vegetables prepared using various cooking methods.

5. Occasional consumption of fish and seafood, mainly the less fatty kinds and those containing less cholesterol.
6. Occasional consumption of seasonal fruits—raw, dried, and cooked.
7. Occasional consumption of a small amount of roasted nuts and seeds.
8. Daily consumption of a small volume of condiments and traditionally prepared seasonings.
9. Daily consumption of an adequate amount of non-stimulating beverages.

Preparation and Eating

1. The processing, preparation, and cooking techniques of foods are to all be traditional methods avoiding application of microwaves and irradiation.
2. Chewing very well is essential; preferably more than 50 times per mouthful is recommended.
3. The use of variety in terms of selection of grains, beans, vegetables, sea vegetables, and other food substances is recommended.
4. Refrain from over-eating and eating before sleeping.

Lifestyle

1. Shift to a more orderly lifestyle from chaotic living.
2. Maintain an orderly environment avoiding disorderly, dark, and depressing surroundings.
3. Engage in active exercise and maintain energetic daily living.
4. Regulate sexual behavior avoiding multiple partners.
5. Cultivate more positive, ambitious wishes towards life.
6. Be grateful to parents, ancestors, people, society, nature and the universe.

7.   Develop the spirit of mutual assistance to brotherhood and sisterhood extended to society at large.

Modern approaches to health and sickness lack a common principle and understanding. Since they lack a common thread that unifies their theory and practice, they often appear contradictory.

In addition, most health approaches are the exclusive domain of health professionals—including experts and specialists—and require special knowledge and training. However, the solution to sickness must be shared by the persons who are directly experiencing it, namely patients and their families. This is especially true with modern degenerative diseases—including cancer and heart disease—that are increasingly associated with the dietary and lifestyle choices that individuals make.

In reality, all health issues rest upon the foundation of daily life, including dietary habits and environmental conditions; factors that each of us must assume personal responsibility for.   Unless we reflect upon our daily patterns of living and revise, improve, and refine them, we will be unable to discover fundamental solutions to the health issues that confront us.

In order to develop a medicine for humanity, we must urgently develop an understanding of the order of the universe, nature, and life. And we need to develop a very practical and simple approach to daily life which everyone can understand and practice. All approaches to health and well-being—ancient and modern, conventional and alternative, physical and psychological, and artificial and natural—can be unified and synthesized under the principles and laws of the order of the universe, which is the order of life and nature itself. With this understanding, each person can share in the creation of a healthful lifestyle.

Over the last fifteen years, macrobiotic education has pioneered the development of a comprehensive approach to human health. In the 1970s, the East West Foundation sponsored regular seminars on the "Principles and Practice of Oriental Medicine" in Boston. Hundreds of doctors, nurses, and other health professionals, along with the general public, participated in these seminars, and gained insight into the traditional macrobiotic health-care practices of Asian countries, and the possibility of integrating these methods in modern practice. Also during that decade, we began yearly conferences on nutritional and macrobiotic approaches to cancer. Numerous health professionals, including cancer researchers, participated in these conferences. The conference proceedings were recorded and published and distributed to leading cancer research centers and public health agencies throughout the world.

Recently, we have organized an international network of physicians who practice the macrobiotic way of life and who recommend it as a viable approach to health promotion and disease prevention. The macrobiotic physicians' network intends also to afford participating doctors opportunities for sharing both personal and professional experiences with one another. It hopes to standardize record-keeping procedures with patients opting to practice the macrobiotic way of life as an approach to their particular needs. This documentation will be used for observing changes and therefore will produce more scientifically oriented data.

This macrobiotic association of physicians, together with the Kushi Foundation, is coordinating seminars for doctors, the first of which was held in March 1987 in Boston. The Kushi Foundation has also begun study programs for people in the health professions, including psychologists, nutritionists, and nurses.

Meanwhile, internationally, physicians' study programs have been presented in France, and plans are now being carried out to begin special training programs for doctors and other health professionals in central Africa, in the Congo. Aveline and I visited the Congo in July, 1987, together with a delegation of doctors and researchers, including Martha Cottrell, M.D., Elinor Levy, Ph.D., and Lawrence Kushi, Sc.D. During our visit, sponsored by the government of the Congo, we presented seminars and conferences on the macrobiotic approach to personal and social health, including reports on the macrobiotic/AIDS research mentioned earlier. Several hundred doctors and government officials attended these events. It is our hope that macrobiotics will be able to serve as a possible solution to the epidemic of AIDS and other degenerative conditions that are prevailing in Africa and other third world countries.

Through these and other efforts, all people, including health professionals and the general public, can jointly participate to secure and develop personal and social health. In the future, the medicine of humanity shall guide all people toward a healthy and sound way of life, including proper dietary practice, for the realization of a healthy and peaceful world.

Macrobiotics: An Approach to the Achievement of Health, Happiness, and Harmony

Vivien Newbold, M.D., F.A.C.E.P.

In December, 1983, a close friend was found to have inoperable colon cancer that had spread to the liver. He was given just four to six months to live. Since there was then and at this writing, still is, no known treatment for this disease once it has spread beyond the intestines and since chemotherapy could, at best, offer only a possibility of temporary prolongation of life, he chose not to receive any medical treatment, but instead to try macrobiotics. He and his family followed the macrobiotic diet one hundred percent, without any deviations, and became totally involved in the macrobiotic way of life. Almost every night his wife and son gave him a *shiatsu* massage. Within three months of being on the macrobiotic diet, he began running, and by September of 1984 he ran a half marathon. In November, 1985, a CT scan could find no sign of cancer and his present health is excellent. This is truly astounding in view of the fact that there is only one recorded case of spontaneous regression of metastatic colon cancer.

In light of this spectacular regression from cancer, I began research into macrobiotics in June, 1984. This included: (1) following a number of patients with cancer who had chosen macrobiotics (with or without chemotherapy); (2) questioning as many patients (or relatives) who had sought macrobiotic counseling, for either pancreatic cancer or brain tumor; (3) sending detailed questionnaires to anyone who felt they had a serious illness and had done much better than expected with macrobiotics; and (4) documenting in the appropriate scientific fashion a number of cases of advanced, medically incurable, terminal patients with biopsy-proven cancer who had followed macrobiotics and who had completely recovered from advanced cancer.

The number of patients in this last group is small, and although it does not prove that macrobiotics can bring about recovery from cancer, it indicates that for the patient who cannot be offered hope medically, it is certainly worth a try. Some people may question whether those cases in which the cancer has disappeared may be due to so-called spontaneous regression (i.e. no one knows why the cancer went away), and although this may be possible, the incidence of spontaneous regression is exceedingly rare.[1,2,3] Regression that has lasted many years is even more rare.[4] It would, therefore, appear reasonable that when a number of patients with "spontaneous regression" have all participated in the same program, that program merits further, thorough investigation.

Too often, macrobiotics is viewed solely as a diet. This is incorrect, because it encompasses every aspect of one's life. Its purpose is to bring every aspect of one's life into balance. To recover from advanced illness, people must do more than just change their diet. They must make radical changes in other areas of their lives. In this chapter, I will describe the major changes in thinking, diet, exercise, and family interaction which I recommend for recovery from advanced illness.

Changes in Thinking

Increasingly, through large prospective studies, psychologists have been able to define the characteristics of people suffering from different illnesses.[5,6] In the case of cancer, for example, the work of Roshan, later confirmed by longitudinal studies done at John Hopkins University, revealed that more than 70 percent of cancer patients in early childhood have true or perceived feelings of rejection by one or both parents. In adult life, cancer patients tend to have difficulty expressing their emotions and in forming deep emotional bonds. Usually, they invest all of their feelings in one love object. This could be a spouse, a child or even work or a hobby. In most cases, approximately one to one-and-a-half years prior to the onset of symptoms, there is a deterioration in that person's relationship with the love object. Thereafter, the person slowly self-destructs.

As Dr. Carl Simonton has described in his book *Getting Well Again*,[7] cancer patients typically become depressed or overwhelmed by hopelessness. However, since they are masters at repressing their negative feelings and putting on a cheerful front, they frequently are not aware of these feelings.

What can be done if one is such a person or is close to such a person? It seems clear to me that more than anything else, cancer patients have a desperate need for unconditional love and acceptance, including unconditional love and approval of themselves. Rev. Louise L. Hay's book, *You Can Heal Your Life*,[8] is exceptionally helpful in understanding and achieving this kind of self-acceptance. In the following paragraphs, I shall outline possible ways to achieve an accepting, loving attitude toward oneself and others.

Gratitude for all things is a cornerstone of macrobiotics. So often, we waste our lives complaining or wishing we could be someone else. If, instead, we repeatedly express gratitude for those very things we complain about and are willing to learn and to make appropriate changes, our whole perspective will change. Suddenly, problems will be seen as challenges which, when met, will produce infinite joy. I would like to share with you a minor problem I had once.

After two months of overindulging in macrobiotic cookies, nuts, and other rich foods, a small lump developed in my left breast. Initially, I was shocked, terrified and angry. Was this lump going to turn out to be a cancer to pay me back for all my bad habits? After obtaining a mammogram which indicated that the possibility of cancer was very remote and seeking macrobiotic counseling, I went on a strict diet. The lump disappeared; however, whenever I overindulged in rich food, the lump would reappear and be very painful. For the first few months, I was angry and resentful. I could not overindulge in the foods I enjoyed so much without a rude reminder from this wretched little thing. Then, one day, I woke up and realized how precious that lump was. It was my warning light which signaled that I was really harming myself. Thereafter, I began to say to myself, many times each day, "Thank you, little lump, for everything you're teaching me. I am happy to learn and ready to change."

Several months later, I came across Rev. Louise Hay's book,

You Can Heal Your Life. Adapting one of her paragraphs, I began saying many times each day, "I love myself. Therefore, I lovingly nourish my body only with the foods my body needs, and my body lovingly responds with radiant health, beauty, flexibility and boundless energy." Although I still overindulge too frequently, those times are becoming fewer and fewer and the degree to which I indulge is becoming less and less. This problem of mine is miniscule compared to that of people dying from a terminal illness, but I have often found that the same basic factors apply. They hate their bodies for becoming ill and their "self-talk" is angry, resentful, and fearful.

Another cornerstone of macrobiotic thinking is that we should take full responsibility for having created *everything*, positive and negative, that happens to us, including our illnesses, accidents, tension within relationships, winning the lottery, and so on. The major difference between modern medicine, as it is currently practiced, and Oriental medicine is not the sciences on which they are based, but the context in which they are practiced. Today, in general, the modern physician sees the patient as an innocent victim of circumstances largely beyond the patient's control and, with few exceptions, the physician pays little attention to the source of the problem. The responsibility for fixing the problem lies largely with the physician, who does the thinking. All the patient has to do is to behave as a helpless, mindless victim and follow instructions.

This attitude is taken in the West to apply to every aspect of one's life. Whenever something goes wrong, people look around to try to find someone else to blame. For example, in my work as an emergency physician, when I ask a teenager, "How did you get this cut?" he or she often replies, "The door hit me," instead of, "I walked into the door and cut myself." In the same vein, people look for others, whether it be a doctor, priest, husband, or macrobiotic counselor, to take responsibility for their lives. One hears patients say, "I put myself in the hands of the very finest physicians in the country." Essentially, the person has abandoned responsibility for himself and given that responsibility to someone else. The majority of sick people come to macrobiotics thinking that all they need to do is eat certain foods to recover—in other words, simply follow a more complex set of instructions. They attempt to dump the responsibility for their recovery on a macrobiotic counselor, as they would a physician, and mindlessly chew the foods. What they need to do is assume responsibility both for having created their illness and for overcoming it.

Macrobiotics views illness as originating from and created by the individual, and in macrobiotics, each individual is completely and solely responsible for his or her own circumstances. All people I have met who have overcome a major illness have taken full responsibility for their illness, have gained an in-depth understanding of their problem, and have taken charge of their life. In many cases, though, the person is too sick initially to make the crucial decisions necessary in a terminal illness, such as whether or not chemotherapy is advisable. In such cases, the family temporarily may take loving and compassionate charge of the decision making, *with the patient's full knowledge*. Then, when the patient has regained strength and judgment, he or she can regain control of decisions. By this, I do not mean the despicable and frequently practiced method of hiding the prognosis from the sick person. This terrible approach, practiced by so many relatives who feel that the pathetic, sick person will be too upset and unable to handle the bad news appropriately, denies them of:

1. *The great privilege of many serious illnesses.* This privilege lies in the realization that modern medicine can do absolutely nothing to cure them of the problem. At best, it can offer only temporary alleviation of symptoms, along with a menagerie of side effects. This realization has mobilized many wonderful people, such as Norman Cousins, Nathan Pritikin, Anthony Sattilaro, Elaine Nussbaum and others to understand, appreciate, and recover from their illnesses.

2. *The time to put their affairs in order.* One of the great advantages of some terminal illnesses, such as cancer, is that it gives people time to put their affairs in order, do some things they have always wanted to do, and make peace with themselves before passing on.

3. *Peace, trust, and open communication in their final hours.*
   I have met many terrified, isolated patients who look on
   in wide-eyed horror, frequently too afraid to ask their
   doctors and relatives any questions regarding their illness.
   They know that, if they did, they would receive only lies.
   The relatives of these patients often rush around with an
   air of busy superiority, whispering at the patient's door
   with their physicians and friends. They are totally in-
   sensitive to the fear, anxiety, and horrifying isolation they
   are creating in their zeal to hide the worst from the patient.

A third cornerstone of macrobiotics, which is not sufficiently
emphasized, is positive self-talk. Positive self-talk is the ultimate
form of taking responsibility for what goes on in one's own
mind and what one creates by one's thinking. Every major illness
I know of is associated with anger, fear, depression, guilt, hopelessness, or other negative emotions. If we listen carefully to the
conversations of people with serious illnesses, we will hear that
the overwhelming thrust of their speech is negative, critical, and
complaining. Occasionally, despite a very serious illness, particularly cancer, patients put on a very good front and are sur-
prisingly jovial and positive, but when we watch them carefully,
particularly their eyes, we see that underneath this facade lie
deeply hidden anger, depression, or other negative emotions.
Sometime these feelings are so deeply repressed that the person
is unaware of them. Changing the constant flow of negative self-
talk and thinking is not easy, but I believe it constitutes a major
factor in turning around a patient's condition.

In order to learn how to do positive self-talk, I would recommend:

1. *Reading the following books*:
   Louise Hays, *You Can Heal Your Life*
   Carl O. Simonton, *Getting Well Again*
   Murphy, *The Power of Your Unconscious Mind*

2. *Writing out and repeating affirmations.*
   I think it is very helpful to write out between ten to twenty
   affirmations about oneself, ranging from statements such

as, "I joyously cook delicious meals that bring radiant health and joy to my family and myself," to statements such as, "I am working in a job that I enjoy doing, and that uses my creative powers." All affirmations must be written and repeated in the present tense. They should be said (out loud or silently) as often as possible and, as we are saying these affirmations, we should feel what it is like when that affirmation is fulfilled. For example, in the above affirmation, "I joyously cook delicious meals that bring radiant health and joy to my family and myself," we should see ourselves joyously cooking, see our family enjoying the food, hear them saying how delicious it is, and see how radiantly healthy they are. Affirmations can be repeated when taking a shower, brushing teeth, walking, waiting in line, driving, and especially when listening to music.

3. *Using guided imagery, or self-hypnosis.*
   In every conceivable group, from Olympic athletes to astronauts walking on the moon,[9] experts are advocating imagery to achieve excellence. I strongly urge imagery to attain excellence in turning problems into triumphs and disease into health. In imagery, people take a moment to create a full sensory picture of what they want to accomplish. It is similar to an affirmation, but affirmations gain their strength by being relatively short and to the point, and they are repeated many times daily. In some circumstances, people find it difficult to visualize what they and their lives would be like if their goal were achieved. In those cases, it is helpful for them to repeat their affirmed goal until it finally becomes believable and they are able to create the full sensory picture or image of fulfillment. The more fully a person can see, hear, feel and taste the image, the stronger the power of imagery becomes. Some people have great difficulty learning to image, and for them it may be helpful to see an expert in self-hypnosis.

4. *Meditating.*
   In meditating, we set aside the time to relax deeply. Then, we may either allow our minds to wander or concentrate

deeply on a full sensory picture of the fulfillment of our goal. By being in a relaxed state, the image becomes more powerful. During a state of deep relaxation, it is possible to ask an *inner guide** to answer questions. This is, in my view, the most interesting and delightful aspect of meditating. There is a glorious world full of surprises to be found when searching within one's mind. I invite you to experiment with different forms of meditatation and see which one you enjoy the most. The art of meditation requires instruction and Simonton's book, *Getting Well Again*, is helpful in this regard.

Diet

The evidence linking diet and the major degenerative diseases affecting modern man is becoming stronger each day, and in areas such as cardiovascular medicine, it is now beyond dispute.[10,11] For those who wish to get up-to-date knowledge of the scientific evidence showing that dietary change can alter the prognosis in established degenerative diseases, including cancer, osteoporosis, atherosclerosis, cardiac disease, high blood pressure, diabetes, arthritis, and urinary disease, I would urge you to read *McDougall's Medicine*.[12] However, although those in the forefront of modern nutritional knowledge can help people overcome many illnesses, macrobiotics is the only diet responsible for a large number of anecdotal recoveries from a wide variety of illnesses, many of which are medically incurable.

For a long time, the medical profession has turned a deaf ear to the role of nutrition in recovery. Despite numerous anecdotal cases of recovery from advanced illness with macrobiotics, there has been until recently no scientific documentation of those recoveries. At the time of this writing, I am preparing an article for a medical journal documenting seven cases of complete regression

---

* *inner guide*—While in the mediative state, some people are able to create inner guides or inner energies that can advise them in different ways.

from advanced, medically incurable cancer. Even though seven cases does not sound like a large number, it is spectacular in view of the extreme rarity of spontaneous regression from advanced cancer.

If one wants to be radiantly healthy, it makes only common sense to follow the healthiest diet one can. Macrobiotics gives people far more than just a diet; it gives them the tools to discover the power of different foods so that they gain the self-mastery to know what to eat to attain their goal. Anyone steeped in Western culture who reads this for the first time may have the same reaction I did initially, "That's a load of bunkum." However, I invite you to try macrobiotics for two to three months, eating the "standard macrobiotic diet," and then go out and eat a pint of ice cream. You will know very quickly what the effects of ice cream are on the body and mind. The optimum diet is unique to each individual, and it is a fascinating adventure finding out what is right for oneself.

This valuable and fascinating kind of experiment is a luxury, however, not available to the person facing imminent death from disease. It is essential that a person in this situation see an experienced teacher and follow their suggestions absolutely accurately. All the people I know of who have overcome a terminal illness have followed their diet extremely carefully, *without any deviations*, until their disease was well behind them. From my research, I can say clearly that those people who indulge in other foods or who feel they know better than macrobiotics and take vitamins in addition to macrobiotics do not do well. After a person has no sign of the disease for at least one year, the patient can deviate occasionally, but macrobiotics must remain the regular daily diet if health is to be maintained. There are many people whose cancers have gone away completely while on a macrobiotic diet only to return when they either: (1) went off the macrobiotic diet completely, or (2) ate predominantly those macrobiotic foods reserved for occasional treats.

If patients are to recover using macrobiotics, the cooking must be accurate. I am frequently amazed at those patients who try to overcome a serious illness and do not take cooking lessons. It is not possible to gain the necessary, thorough understanding of macrobiotic cooking from cookbooks. It requires numerous lessons from a variety of cooking teachers. Ideally, both the patients and their spouses, children, parents, grandchildren and loving friends should accompany them to cooking lessons. However, during the height of the sense of crisis in the illness and until the patients are well on the road to recovery, it is better for someone else—spouse, child, parent, grandchild, loving friend —to cook for them. (This will be discussed in greater detail in the next section, "The Family.")

Some patients feel that they do not have time to learn to cook macrobiotically, so they merely bring in a hired cook or pick up take-out meals. With few exceptions, such people do not do well. First, they never gain a real understanding of macrobiotics and second, they rarely receive the energy that comes from food that has been prepared by someone who loves them. To someone foreign to macrobiotics, this idea may sound absurd, but it is a significant factor in recovery. Although each of us is different, developing sensitivity to the energy in food usually takes at least one to two years. To help someone recover from advanced illness, the food should be cooked with love, with sensitivity only to the needs of the sick person, and with a strong positive expectation of the person's recovery.

In line with this, I always advise sick people trying macrobiotics *not to travel for at least a year after their illness is well behind them.* The reasons for this are:

1. Each diet is in harmony with the person's environment. Sudden changes in the environment result in necessary changes in the diet which, although small, may be of great importance. Patients are not yet sensitive enough to their body's needs to make these minor adjustments in their diet.

2. Sudden changes in the environment lead to a "jolt" in the body's careful balance. We all get disproportionately tired when we travel. A person's body that is struggling to overcome a disease process cannot tolerate such a jolt.

3.   Some people seem to think they can travel and pick up take-out meals as they go. This is fine for those in good health, but for the ailing, they are unlikely to find take-out food that is prepared just for their problem. Also, it may be difficult to resist a special dessert or deep-fried dish which may be included in the take-out dinner, but which is not recommended for their condition.

4.   It is extremely difficult for people to cook while traveling. If it is absolutely necessary, however, patients should take their own cook with them.

Many people are extremely concerned about the weight loss that sometimes occurs when one first eats macrobiotically. If it is true that the macrobiotic diet allows the body to rid itself of accumulated toxins, then it is only reasonable that, initially, there could be weight loss, particularly if the person was overweight to begin with. In some cases, people dip below their ideal weight, and later regain weight to their optimal level. Unfortunately, some people remain below their optimum weight, becoming painfully thin and rigid. They can appear sullen and depressed and look and behave jaundiced with the world. In my experience, the major reasons for this occurrence are:

1.   *Excessive consumption of salt.*   Salt plays a critical role in the macrobiotic diet, yet excessive use of it results in marked rigidity, accelerated weight loss, a constant craving for more food, and an overwhelming desire for sweets and oil. In the experience of Geraldine Walker, one of the finest macrobiotic healing cooks, excess salt slows the healing process and delays the elimination of toxins.

2.   *Lack of leafy greens.*   Leafy greens can be difficult to obtain and take time to clean. Many people coming from a Western diet do not like the taste of leafy green vegetables. Some of the healing greens can be tough to chew or taste bitter unless cooked with ingenuity and care. By

cutting them into small pieces, or by mixing the bitter vegetables with sweet vegetables, such as onions, the greens can be a very enjoyable part of the meal.

3. *Excessive consumption of oil.* Oil has been shown to (1) cause clumping of red blood cells as they flow through the blood vessels, (2) decrease the oxygen carrying capacity of the blood by twenty percent, and (3) on a chronic basis produce a change in the blood brain barrier.[13] A person who awakes bounding with energy and sits down to a large breakfast of pancakes, butter, honey, sausages and eggs will, by the end of this oil-rich meal, usually feel bogged down and only have the energy to go back to bed. Health food cookies baked with oil, flour and sweeteners are fine when eaten occasionally, but on a regular basis, they can have a detrimental effect on a person's metabolism.

4. *Coffee in excess.* Coffee has an excitatory effect on the body and in large amounts can create imbalance.

5. *Cigarettes.* The extremely deleterious effects of cigarette smoking on health are well established. Smoking is no part of the macrobiotic diet, and macrobiotics does not render one immune to its devastating effects, just as it does not render one immune to the effects of ice cream. Among other things, smoking results in an immediate and marked decrease in the blood supply to the brain and can thus dull the thinking.

6. *Lack of exercise.* Many individuals who become thin and rigid after changing their diet get no exercise, fresh air or sunshine. People are meant to do vigorous physical exercise in the fresh air and they cannot come into physical and mental harmony without it.

7. *Eating too rigidly.* Some people eat rigidly, by the book without reflection. We should ask if the way we are eating

is creating radiant health, happiness, and flexibility of mind and body. Rigidity of eating often leads to arrogance.

8. *Negative thinking.* One of the real traps that people can fall into is negative thinking, especially guilt. It is easy for people to feel guilty for not eating and chewing properly, or to feel anger about their past. It is easy for people to find themselves thinking, "If only I cooked better, then everything would be fine," or "If only I chewed better, my life would go well," and so on. Many of us are caught in this trap, as well as in the trap of judging others who do not eat as strictly ("He's not really macrobiotic. I saw him eat a croissant."), or in the trap of resenting those who eat enormous amounts of junk food and yet suffer no apparent ill effects. Louise Hay's book, *You can Heal Your Life*, can be very helpful in this respect. It can help us realize that negative self-talk like "I'm not good enough" or "If only I could do this better, then I would be good enough" has an extremely deleterious effect, not only on our health, but on every aspect of our lives. I believe firmly that illness, any illness, is due primarily to a combination of poor diet and negative self-talk. It is through changing these that miracles can begin to happen.

Beside the thin, rigid person trying to eat macrobiotically, there is another group of people who do not appear radiantly healthy. Instead of being rigid and jaundiced, however, these people appear sallow, limp, and may be either too thin or too plump. This problem was brought home to me fully the first year I was macrobiotic. Then and now, my chief goal was to be a sweet, gentle wife, so I decided not to eat any fish whatsoever. At first I felt better, but after about six months, I began to feel increasingly weak and limp. I craved some food that would give me a spark of energy. I found myself eating peanut butter and jam in large amounts. Instead of giving me energy, the nuts and sweets gave me a headache and made me feel stuck. I kept trying different cooking techniques, all to no avail.

Finally, I could hardly get out of bed in the morning. Instead of being a sweet, gentle wife, I was dull, whiny and constantly complaining, as I moped around the house. At last I became fascinated by fish. I wanted very much to feel like a strong salmon swimming upstream and bounding over the waterfalls. I dreamed about it night after night, and I got Herman Aihara's book, *Learning from Salmon*, in the hope of finding the answer there. Finally, the penny dropped. I needed some fish. I discovered that a small amount of fish was right for me, given my state of health, the work I do, and the lifestyle I lead. If I eat too much, I become excessively aggressive and have nightmares. As time passes, and my body is becoming increasingly accustomed to whole grains and beans, I find I need less and less fish, and if I eat too much fish, I feel out of balance.

Most people, whether macrobiotic or not, find it much easier to keep their diet and themselves in balance when they exercise vigorously. Exercising in the fresh outdoors is especially beneficial. It is not only mentally more stimulating, as it puts people in closer touch with nature, but it is also much healthier, as pollution can be seventy times higher indoors than outdoors. The work of Simonton and others has indicated that patients who exercise daily do better than those who do not. If macrobiotics is right, and cancer and other diseases are the accumulation of toxins and other excesses which the body is unable to get rid of, then it seems to make sense that if we burn off more through exercise and excrete more through sweat, we may get rid of those toxins a lot faster.

For several reasons, I highly recommend that people use the time that they are exercising to do imaging, as explained earlier. First, imaging while exercising helps to protect the person from the type of negative thinking that can lead to injury. If the exercisers resent and resist the exercise and say to themselves, "I hate running. I'm just doing this awful running so that I can stay slim. I wish I were home in bed," they are much more likely to incur an injury so that they can no longer exercise. Second, imaging while exercising transforms the previously unpleasant program of exercise into one which can gradually become extremely enjoyable. For example, if while running, people repeatedly see themselves as slim, beautiful, handsome, radiantly happy, and succeeding in all aspects of their lives, then they return home feeling triumphant, revitalized, and confident. Third, it has been well established that prolonged and vigorous exercise can lead to a state in which the body releases endorphins. Endorphins are morphine-like compounds which lead to the so-called runner's high. It is during these times that imaging is especially powerful.

The purpose of macrobiotics is to gain self-mastery of every aspect of our lives. We must reflect daily on our way of life and on the effects of the food we have eaten. When we eat something, we ask ourselves, "How do I feel, more cloudy or more clear, more stable or more jittery, more energetic or more stuck, more loving to myself and the world or more critical and aggressive?" and so on. We do this not so that we become preoccupied with food, but so that we can gain a clearer insight into how to eat to realize our goals. Initially, we need to follow the guidance of a fine macrobiotic instructor, but as time passes and our intuition and understanding of food grows, we discover what is right for each one of us. One of the major hurdles we must overcome is knowing the difference between needing to eat something— knowing that it is right for us today—and wanting to eat something because it tastes good. I have found the following adaptation of Louise Hay's work most helpful and I say it to myself many times each day, particularly before going food shopping, cooking and eating:

"I love myself; therefore, I take loving care of my body. I lovingly nourish it only with the foods and beverages it needs, I lovingly groom it and dress it, and my body lovingly responds with vibrant health and energy."

The Family

All crises are times of great opportunity, since it is under such circumstances that people are most willing to change. A time of crisis is a time for careful reflection by all concerned, for re-evaluation of every aspect of one's life, and for redirection. Every illness, one's own as well as that of a family member, is a crisis, a clear sign that we are doing something wrong and that re-evaluation and changes are needed.

The vast majority of people think that when one member of a family becomes ill, it is entirely the problem of the sick person and has nothing to do with anyone else. They see the patient as a helpless, unlucky victim, struck down by unknown forces. They view their own role, at best, as one of being sympathetic and kind. This pathetic approach to disease and, for many people, to most aspects of their lives, leaves them powerless, blowing like a leaf in the winds of fate.

Macrobiotics offers the possibility of self-mastery and power in the face of disease. It invites people to take full responsibility for every aspect of their life. It is in this context that each family member must take full responsibility for the well-being of all the other members of the family, *not through control*, but through action, behavior and thinking. This is the meaning of family support, and in my view, it is the single most significant factor in a patient's recovery. Thus, if a husband, wife, child, parent or close friend is sick, in order for that person to recover, we must recognize that we and our entire family are sick, both in mind and body, and that we are responsible for that illness.

We should inquire into all the different ways in which we have caused that illness, even though this may initially cause us to feel guilty. We can move guilt to a feeling of power over the problem by taking the steps necessary for recovery. When we take such a stand, we move from the comfortable, wishy-washy attitude of complaining and blaming others for our circumstance to an adventure fraught with difficult challenges, for which the rewards are limitless. The following paragraphs outline the major actions which people can take if they are a relative or close friend of a seriously ill person.

Relatives or close friends of a seriously ill person need to express gratitude to the sick person for becoming ill. Through their illness they have been forced to reflect and they have realized that they themselves were headed for self-destruction and that the illness has allowed them to change and help themselves. They need to show the patient by all their actions that their recovery to radiant health and happiness takes precedence over all else in their lives. They cannot just give lip service to this. They need to think only in terms of the patient's recovery and their loving actions should reflect this constantly.

Additionally, relatives or close friends of a seriously ill person need to follow the patient's diet one-hundred percent as though they themselves had the disease.* A seriously ill person invariably feels isolated, alone, and confused. When the sick person eats food which is different from the rest of the family, it increases his or her feelings of isolation.

Imagine for a moment how much it means to most of us to sit down and share food, the same food from the same pot, with our family and friends. If we see ourselves as sick and frightened, sitting and eating our own plate of food, which no one wants to share with us, we are trapped there with our food, unable to enjoy those familiar dishes which the rest of our family is eating. We can smell the rich aromas that remind us so much of eating with our family as a child, and we want to reach out and eat with everyone else, just the way we used to, so that we can be a part of things again and forget that we are dying.

We take a little bite believing that maybe it won't hurt, but if someone says, "You're not supposed to be eating that. Stick to your diet. We want you to live. We care about you," we then feel crushed and guilty ("How could I have been so weak-willed? I'm never going to do this again. I hate myself for it."). Or maybe someone says, "Go on. Have the whole thing. It'll do you good. You've lost a lot of weight." We then feel confused ("What on earth am I doing on this crazy diet anyway? Why am I torturing myself like this?"). Day after day, meal after meal, scenes like these are repeated. When the vast majority of families behave like this, it is not surprising that many people do not recover, and that some people even die faster.

By eating the sick patient's diet with him one-hundred percent, the family accomplishes many extremely important things. First, it makes that family a team whose goal is radiant health

---

* Of course, individual modifications in diet are required for each person.
—*Editor*

and happiness for each member. Second, it lets the sick person know that each family member believes in macrobiotics and feels that they too were headed for serious illness. Thus, the sick person, instead of being a burden, has truly benefitted the entire family. Third, taking responsibility for the disease with the sick person and eating their macrobiotic diet with them one-hundred percent is a dramatic expression of the family's unconditional love, and of their degree of commitment to his or her recovery. Fourth, it is only through eating macrobiotically that one can begin to understand macrobiotics. If the person who cooks for the sick person does not eat macrobiotically one-hundred percent, he or she cooks mechanically and the food does not have the power to heal. By the same token, if an outside macrobiotic cook comes in and cooks for the person, there cannot be the same love, care and understanding of the patient. During the learning phase, hiring a cook is sometimes an option for a few of the meals, but ideally, the family should do almost all of the cooking for the patient. Cooking macrobiotically can be fun for the entire family and, in fact, making it fun and creating an atmosphere of joy within the home makes recovery more likely.

In my experience, patients who cook for themselves generally do not do so well. For them, it is a long, slow haul. We all need someone else's creativity in our food occasionally, and seriously ill people tend to make the same mistakes when cooking macrobiotically, and to put back the same creativity into the food, that made them sick in the first place. It is tragic to see a person trying to cook macrobiotically on their own to recover from serious illness. The path for this valiant man or woman is a long, slow struggle. Occasionally, this may be because the patient complains when other family members cook and make mistakes. It is important for the patient to express appreciation to those who are cooking for him or her.

Whenever someone else cooks for us, we can reflect on how we feel, and we will often be amazed at how much we learn about ourselves and other people. When a meal is cooked just right by a happy person, we feel enlivened, but if the person who cooked was angry and resentful, then the meal will not turn out well, no matter what the experience of the cook, and those eating it will not feel well after it. Thus, we should be very careful about who cooks for us, and when we cook, we should make a point of being joyous and thinking happy thoughts.

There are few better ways to affirm unconditional love for a sick person than by daily giving that person a massage for half-an-hour or an hour, no matter what has gone on during the day. In macrobiotics, the massage usually used is shiatsu massage and it is one in which the *meridians*, or energy lines, of the body are stimulated. Tumors themselves should not be massaged directly, and patients with advanced illnesses should seek advice as to the type of massage which would be most appropriate for them. Courses in shiatsu massage are available at most macrobiotic centers. Shiatsu massage can have a relaxing or energizing effect on the body. Generally speaking, it is not a sexually arousing massage.

Macrobiotics recommends that every morning and evening one rub one's body down vigorously with a hot towel, but it is far better if a family member takes the trouble to do this. If the family member rubs the sick person's body down every night, no matter what, and then gives a shiatsu massage, the sick person will fall into a restful sleep. The hot rubdown and the massage, when given by a loved one, have the effects of relaxing the body and of calming the mind through the dedication and love which the family. member has actively expressed. I firmly believe that massage is essential not only to facilitating recovery from advanced illness but to the establishment of joy, peace, and harmony within the family.

There is now little doubt that the mind plays a role in most disease processes, and there are increasing numbers of people who feel that one's thought patterns are the origins of all diseases and mishaps. The work on mind and immunity leaves little doubt that the immune system is affected by one's thinking. The mental attitude of the patient's entire family is very important. In most cases, the family views the patient as someone whose body is about to collapse, and daily they look at the person for signs of deterioration. Is it surprising, then, that the patient views himself as a disaster waiting to happen?

Macrobiotics asks that every member of the family enter into a spirit of adventure towards total health. When each family member, including the patient, is grateful for the illness and actively visualizes the patient's and the family's recovery to radiant health and boundless joy and energy, the patient views his situation as a challenge. When each family member, again including the patient, visualizes the patient and family as radiantly healthy, joyous and happy, not just three times a day, but during every waking moment, the family enters into a positive spirit of healing instead of one of decay and collapse.

The road from illness to recovery is generally not an easy one and the family will meet many challenges along the way, particularly as the relationships within it heal. Since the patient is not accustomed to unconditional love, unconsciously he or she may repeatedly challenge that love to see if it really is unconditional. In such circumstances, it is often difficult for the family to remain steadfast. Here are several tips which may help. Family members need to:

1. Express gratitude for the problem and tell themselves they are willing to change.

2. Take *full* responsibility for the problem themselves. Making it someone else's responsibility is much more pleasant, but it offers them no power to change the situation.

3. Examine carefully what the pay-off or hidden value of hanging onto the problem has for them. This is usually very difficult and will probably take time to understand. For example, if a family member has had prolonged hostility toward another family member, that has usually resulted in an "I'm right—she's wrong" attitude. The hidden value in such a case can be the sense of self-righteousness and superiority afforded to the person who feels in the right. In order to learn to love unconditionally, each family member can benefit from relinquishing his or her hidden payoff(s) at having the problem.*

* "*The Forum*," a two weekend workshop held in most major cities, can be very helpful to people in bringing about an understanding of the payoffs they are deriving from their problems.

In summary, macrobiotics is far more than a diet. It is a process by which people daily strive to bring every aspect of their lives into balance. Macrobiotics asks that people, in their attitude toward life, be grateful for everything, including the problems they are facing, and that they assume responsibility for creating everything that happens to them. This includes being responsible for their own thinking and self-talk, whether positive or negative, and for the consequences which result from it. The purpose of the macrobiotic study of diet is to give people an understanding of the effects of different foods on the body so that they know how to eat to accomplish their goals. This knowledge provides people with an essential tool in the development of self-mastery. To maintain a well-balanced body and mind, the body must be cared for lovingly not only through diet but also through exercise. For those people who are considering macrobiotics to try to recover from serious medical problems, I recommend that they embrace it in its fullest sense. For such seriously ill people, it is essential that they follow the diet recommended for them by a well-trained macrobiotic teacher absolutely accurately and without any deviations.

Family members and loving friends wishing to support a seriously ill person who has chosen the macrobiotic approach should also embrace every aspect of macrobiotics. By this I mean that they should take full responsibility for creating everything that happens, including the patient's illness. This concept may produce emotional discomfort and guilt, but the reason for assuming this responsibility is to gain empowerment, *not* guilt. People are able to transcend the guilt by realizing that, having created the problem, they therefore have the power to overcome it through positive action. Family members should support the sick person by eating the diet with the patient one-hundred percent, by attending cooking classes and cooking for the sick person, by daily giving the patient a hot rubdown and shiatsu massage, and above all, by giving the patient their unconditional love.

Macrobiotics offers the possibility of triumph over devastating illnesses and of harmony, joy, and peace in every aspect of life!

References

[1] Charles M. Shapiro, "Remission of Metastatic Adenocarcinoma of Colon," *Journal of the American Medical Association*, Nov. 11, 1983, Vol. 250, No. 18.

[2] T. C. Everson and W. H. Cole, *Spontaneous Regression of Cancer* (Philadelphia: Saunders, 1966).

[3] Waren H. Cole, "Efforts to Explain Spontaneous Regression of Cancer," *Journal of Surgical Oncology*, 17: 201–209 (1981).

[4] Ibid.

[5] Larry Sherwitz, et al., "Self-Involvement and the Risk Factors for Coronary Heart Disease," *Advances*, Vol. 2, No. 2. Spring, 1985.

[6] Carl Simonton, *Getting Well Again* (New York: Bantam Books, 1980).

[7] Ibid.

[8] Louise L. Hay, *You Can Heal Your Life* (Santa Monica, CA.: Hay House, 1984).

[9] Dennis E. Waitley, *The Psychology of Winning*, Audio Tapes, Nightingale Conaut Corporation.

[10] *Diet, Nutrition, and Cancer*, American Institute of Cancer Research, Washington, D. C. 20029. (Complimentary copies available on request.)

[11] John McDougall, *McDougall's Medicine: A Challenging Second Opinion* (Piscataway, N. J.: New Century Publishers, Inc., 1985).

[12] Ibid.

[13] C. Cullen, "Intravascular Aggregation and Adhesiveness of the Blood Elements Associated with Elementary Lipemia and Injections of Large Molecular Substances. Effect of Blood Brain Barrier," *Circulation*, 9: 335, 1954.

Cancer Revisited—Seven Years Later

Christiane Northrup, M.D.

Writing this article about cancer has taken me a long time. Seven years ago I was eager to believe that there was a right way and a wrong way to deal with cancer. I now find that I do not believe there is any one answer to the problem.

Back when I first started to suggest macrobiotics to people with cancer, I would close the door before speaking, afraid my colleagues would overhear my heresy to medical doctrine. Over the years the role of diet in healing has become much more widely accepted and I no longer close the door before speaking. I now believe that each illness we have is a message from our deepest self trying to get our attention. The best method of treatment for any given patient depends on what resonates most with that person's belief system about the disease.

In 1986, my colleagues and I created a health-care center called Women to Women. Our intention is to guide people in seeking the message their illness has for them and then help them choose a healing program from among many options.

I am not a primary-care physician for women with cancer. The patients who come to see me are self-selected; they have already chosen the road less traveled. I have a context to offer—a pathway to share that can lead to meaning. It is within that context that I share with you my experience with cancer.

When I wrote *Examining Cancer* in 1980,* I was a year out of my four-year obstetrics and gynecology residency, just beginning my private practice. Though my interest in health-enhancing modalities such as macrobiotics was keen, my actual experience with them was still limited. As I read the article now, I am delighted to find that most of my views have not substantially changed.

---

* Published in *Cancer and Heart Disease: The Macrobiotic Approach to Degenerative Disorders* by Michio Kushi and associates, Japan Publications, 1982.

In 1980, one in four people got cancer in this country. Now, in 1987, the rate is one in three. The orthodox treatment approaches of surgery, chemotherapy and radiation have not changed substantially. Despite reports that we are "winning the war on cancer," the actual statistics are not very comforting. John Cairns of the Harvard School of Public Health writes in *Scientific American*, ". . . apart from the success with Hodgkin's disease, childhood leukemia and a few other cancers, it is not possible to detect any sudden change in death rates for any of the major cancers that could be credited to chemotherapy."

In their article, "Progress Against Cancer," (*New England Journal of Medicine*, May 1986) Drs. Bailar and Smith state, ". . . we are losing the war against cancer, notwithstanding progress against several uncommon forms of the disease, improvements in palliation, and extension of the productive years of life. A shift in research emphasis, from research on treatment to research on prevention, seems necessary if substantial progress against cancer is to be forthcoming."

What About Prevention? Information linking diet and other environmental factors to cancer is increasingly available. The Maine Bureau of Health recently sponsored a symposium entitled "Conference on Cancer Prevention and Control: Setting an Agenda for Maine." The conference goal was to establish a practical plan to decrease cancer incidence by applying what we know about risk factors. Seven years ago when I began lecturing on the link between diet and cancer, this kind of mainstream acceptance was rare. Magazine articles on the subject are now common. Indeed, the American Cancer Society has changed its former stance that diet and cancer are unrelated; encouraging increased consumption of dark green leafy and cruciferous vegetables. A current ad campaign states that "A defense against cancer can be cooked up in your kitchen." But while there is a growing awareness of the diet-cancer connection, one need only survey the menu in any standard American restaurant to see how far we as a nation must go to change to a healthy diet.

What Causes Cancer: No Simple Answers. In *Examining Cancer,* I explored the various theories of cancer causation such as radiation exposure, genetic predisposition and infectious agents. Though each of these factors might be associated with certain cancers, we are unlikely to find precise cause-and-effect models when dealing with a disease as complex as cancer. Many studies, for example, link certain viruses to cancer. Even if a certain virus were implicated in a given cancer, however, we still can not predict how that cancer will behave in a particular individual.

Every individual is unique, with a unique life history, immune system, diet and genetic constitution; these have been called "host factors." Even though statistics give us some idea about what happens in populations, they can be misleading or irrelevant when dealing with an individual. Why two similar people with the identical cancer will often differ dramatically in the course of their cancer treatment has long fascinated many healers and has become the subject of increasing amounts of research recently.

The Exceptional Cancer Patient. Over the years I have had the privilege of sharing in the healing process with a large number of patients. Some have done very well with conventional methods of healing such as drugs and surgery, some have done well with macrobiotics, many have done poorly regardless of their treatment modality.

There is a common thread running through the lives of those who show a strong will to live. Bernie Siegal, M.D., a cancer surgeon, writes about those who survive even "terminal" cancer in his book *Love, Medicine and Miracles.* He uses the adjective "exceptional" to characterize those who "beat the odds," and says that they are always in the minority. For her book, *The Cancer Survivors,* Judith Glassman interviewed a number of people who have survived "terminal cancer" despite well-documented odds to the contrary. The most striking thing about all of these people is that each engineered his or her own recovery and each had an enormous will to live.

Because of my ongoing interest in and interaction with exceptional cancer patients, I have changed my approach to cancer; I no longer suggest one treatment modality over another. I refuse to decide for a given patient what treatment they should have for a given illness. Instead, I know that each person is fully capable, with some guidance, of choosing the methods that will best enhance his or her healing process.

Cancer and Relationship to Time.   In my patients who have been positively transformed by the experience of cancer, I have found that their relationship to time changes. A striking example of this is a fifty-five-year-old woman from northern Maine who was diagnosed with breast cancer in the spring of 1986. She elected to have a lumpectomy with no further treatment other than dietary change. When she came back in the fall looking radiant and healthy, I asked her how her summer had been. She laughed and said, "I rode my horse every day and spent hours roaming through the meadows and woods. Summer hasn't felt like this since I was a kid. It seemed to go on and on and I feel like I took summer into every pore of my body. Oh . . . I also learned to juggle."

This woman has really learned how to live. If we can learn to really BE in life, then time takes on new meaning.

In an article entitled "After Cancer, The Problems of Surviving" by Meredith Maran (*Medical Self Care*, May/June, 1986), a participant in a survivors support group stated, "The hardest part since I've been ill, is trying to keep that special intensity. As awful as being sick was—my life had more meaning that year than it's ever had. I don't want to lose that feeling." The people who continue to thrive after the diagnosis of cancer are, I believe, the ones who can honestly say, "Thank God I had cancer . . . it has changed my whole life."

Our bodies continually provide us with signals that our lives are getting out of balance. These signals may start out as small accidents or minor illnesses. Then, if we fail to pay attention, something comes up to grab that attention. If it takes cancer to get you to take complete stock of your life, embrace it. You might consider giving up the stance of "fighting" your cancer as if it is something separate from you. How about creating a dialogue with it to find out what lesson it has for you before bidding it farewell? I realize that this concept is paradoxical: on the one hand you must work hard to overcome cancer, and at the same time you must transcend the illusion that it is the enemy. Both are true. Dr. Elizabeth Kubler-Ross says, "If one is in pain, comfort must be sought. The body is asking for something. Don't keep denying it." Cancer comes when we have denied our soul's needs again and again.

Guidelines

A Word of Caution.   Many people expect their illness to be treated as quickly and painlessly as driving through McDonald's for breakfast. For those interested in natural treatments, this approach takes the form of "What vitamins should I take?" or "What special food should I be eating?" Though taking vitamins and eating certain foods may be an improvement over past habits, this approach still represents a dualistic "parts" mentality rather than a "whole systems" or truly holistic approach.

Diet.   Of all the dietary systems daily put forth as "the answer," only macrobiotics is a true whole-systems approach. In deciding what is best to eat, macrobiotic philosophy addresses where you live, what your daily activities are like, and what you want to do with your life. It is also concerned with the food quality— both substantial and subtle. Who grew it? Where? Who cooked it? How? All of these things make a difference.

The unifying principle of yin and yang has always impressed me with its inherent common sense, simplicity and beauty. In its most expansive sense, macrobiotics is, of course, much more than a diet.

As a diet, and as a healing modality in particular, I have never seen another system capable of improving people's facial features so quickly. Within only one to two months after changing from the standard American diet to this way of eating, people often become strikingly more attractive.

The Addictive Process.   After seven years of recommending macrobiotics, I have come to the realization that very few people are capable of making significant dietary changes. Why is it so hard for people to change their eating patterns? The answer, I believe, lies in the addictive process. Without understanding this, one can never give dietary advice that stands a chance of being put into practice by more than a very few.

It is estimated that 75 percent of American women have eating disorders ranging from anorexia on the one hand to bulimia and compulsive overeating on the other. Ninety-six percent of overweight people who lose weight gain it back within a year. Anne Wilson Schaef, in her latest book *When Society Becomes An Addict*, divides addictions into two major categories: substance addictions and process addictions. She points out that both function in essentially the same way and are quite common in our culture, as are multiple addictions. She defines substance, or "ingestive," addictions as "addictions to substances," usually artificially refined or produced, that are deliberately taken into the body. Refined, processed food is itself an addictive substance. As Schaef points out, "Treating food addictions can be especially difficult since food is essential to life and the addict cannot withdraw from it completely in order to recover. . . ." She goes on, "One can be addicted to eating, to not eating, or to eating a huge quantity of food and then desperately trying to get rid of it." Those with eating disorders often speak of "stuffing" their feelings with food.

Schaef writes, "An addiction keeps us unaware of what is going on inside us. We do not have to deal with our anger, pain, depression, confusion, or even our joy and love, because we do not feel them, or we feel them only vaguely. In time, this lack of *internal* awareness deadens our internal processes, which in turn allows us to remain addicted." Denial that there is a problem, be it an excess intake of alcohol, food or work, is the hallmark of all addictions. Denial goes a long way toward explaining how we continue to consume the standard American high-fat, low-nutrient diet despite all the mounting evidence that it is contributing to so many of our most common and serious health problems.

Lynn Andrews, author and medicine woman, has said that all addictions exist to keep us from getting in touch with our true selves. Schaef suggests that our recovery from addiction comes when we begin to move into a "living process" system in which we honor ourselves and our deepest knowing. Getting in touch with that long denied "knowing" is the process of recovery.

Getting Started. Having the diagnosis of cancer often motivates people quickly to make changes that can enhance the quality of life. It really pulls our attention to what is important. So how do you get to the point where you prefer broccoli to Big Macs and pizza? First, be willing to accept the fact that you have a choice over what you eat. No one is a victim. At first it seems inconvenient to choose whole foods, but it is also inconvenient to have heart disease, cancer and excess body fat. Once you make a change, the taste buds gradually change so that going back to the old "Standard American Diet" (S.A.D.) is simply unacceptable. After a while, you no longer like that food and/or your body reacts to it in ways that are unpleasant soon after eating it.

For starters, I recommend the following:

- A two-week period of whole foods—ideally a personalized macrobiotic diet to "cleanse the intuition."
- If possible, hire a skilled cook or have a friend or family member attend cooking classes to learn how to prepare the food. When one is sick, it is best not to try learning a whole new way of cooking without support.
- Consider attending a residential program such as that offered by the Kushi Foundation in the Berkshires. Learning is always easier when done in community. And, being with others who are also healing will often enhance your own recovery.

The two-week trial run I suggest gives the body adequate time to start noticing the healing effects of whole foods. Over and over, people return to my office following dietary change saying, "I never would have believed that diet could make this much difference in how I feel." Yet, the addictive nature of devitalized food remains very real and despite good results people often slide back into the eating patterns set in childhood. You can break free of these old habits if you love yourself enough to take the time to eat well.

Food is important to healing because, as John McDougall, M.D. points out, "Molecule for molecule, food is our largest contact with the environment." I am continually astounded by how much time and energy people will spend "dancing around in the aura" without changing their physical vibrations through food change. We are spiritual beings experiencing life in a physical world. Eating is part of this reality.

Beyond Diet. All great spiritual and healing traditions have stressed the role of diet in healing; but to focus too intently on diet sometimes means missing the overwhelming stresses that, I believe, set the stage for cancer. To tell a woman with breast cancer that her "too yin" diet is the sole cause of her problem when she lives with an alcoholic husband and had an alcoholic or abusive father is not always entirely helpful, nor is it holistic.

Food is only one part of the healing equation. We must make some balance between being paranoid about every bite and blessing every bite. Water that has been prayed over is different from ordinary water and the effects of diet are tremendously influenced by one's state of consciousness. Try simply BEING with food in a compassionate way.

I realize there is a paradox here. When one begins macrobiotics for *recovery* from a particular condition, the dietary regimen must be followed precisely for a while. This holds true for any healing modality; one must be committed to it if one has chosen it because commitment to a healing modality reflects commitment to oneself. Value yourself enough to give your regimen time to work; the very energy of your commitment is a large part of the healing process.

Guilt Versus Responsibility. If you have cancer, do not beat yourself up. Wayne Dyer, Ph.D., in his popular book *Your Erroneous Zones* states, "Guilt is immobilization in the present over something that happened in the past." Take responsibility for your health by actively participating in the healing process. Responsibility means ability to respond. Far too many people are content to hand their lives over to someone else.

Self-Love. I often ask my patients to practice self-love and self-acceptance by looking straight at themselves in the mirror each morning and stating, "I accept myself unconditionally right now." If that is difficult to do, they especially need to do it. And I write the phrase on a prescription blank for added impact; it is good medicine. After about thirty days, something happens and that self-acceptance becomes a reality.

Love of self requires that we practice seeing our individual magnificence daily. Just as there are no two snowflakes alike, there are no two humans alike. Planet Earth has never seen the likes of you before, nor will there be another you again. This is really quite astounding—and is cause for celebration. All of us would do well to learn how to receive graciously the gifts offered to us. To do this is not selfish, though there is much confusion about this issue. We simply cannot give when our own cup is empty. To continue giving when one feels depleted results in resentment and further depletion.

Exercise and Bodywork. Some type of exercise is a necessary adjunct to healing. Whether it be dancing, walking, tai-chi, or a combination of these, please know that your body, though it may be in pain now, was designed to move and to give you pleasure. In addition, the increased oxygenation of tissues that comes with exercise and deep breathing helps rid the body of the anaerobic environment that favors the growth of cancer. Our studies of psychoneuroimmunology have begun to document the optimal hormonal and immune states associated with happiness, fulfillment and pleasure.

In Ashley Montagu's book *Touching, The Human Significance of the Skin*, the need for close and frequent human contact is beautifully documented. The type of cuddling that is usually reserved for children would enhance the lives of all of us. Try a daily foot or back rub and then work into some type of full body massage such as *shiatsu*.

Doing What Comes Naturally. What is it you have always wanted to do but have been putting off "until you had the time?" *DO IT NOW.* The art of creating that which you love, be it a painting, a trip, or a relationship, has extraordinary healing power.

Lawrence LeShan, in his book *You Can Fight For Your Life,* says that the key question for cancer patients to ask is not "How did I get my cancer and how can I get rid of it?" but "What is the unique song that I'm supposed to be singing in my life?" What is the gift you would leave Planet Earth? Would you plant gardens? Would you learn to tap dance? Try to remember what you loved to do when you were about age nine or ten, and that should give you some clues if you are currently out of touch with your Self.

When a Family Member Has Cancer. I can not begin to count how many times I have been called by a family member asking me to please, "Talk to mother—tell her about macrobiotics—you're a doctor, she'll listen to you." In my naive early days as a doctor, I used to think that making such calls was not only helpful but was, in fact, my duty. However, individuals who have cancer must choose the approach they wish to pursue. Serious illness can be a time of intense healing for the patient and can also be a time of intense healing within the family. To accomplish this healing, we must stop trying to control the process.

We must be honest with each other. Realize that when we withhold information from one another in the guise of "protecting" the other person, we are denying that person his full human capacity of self-determination. The greatest gift we can give to another is that of our full unconditional presence. That means getting rid of our need to control, please, or manipulate.

When one is not honest with another human being, when necessary information is not shared, the other person knows it. We are born with the capacity to sense the truth. I have found that people deal with the truth, lovingly presented, much more gracefully than is generally imagined.

Inner Knowing. Ultimately, to be cured we must embrace the message the disorder has brought to our consciousness. We must also access our inner truth about our needs. The old adage, "To thine own self be true; then thou can be false to no man," was never more applicable than in the case of cancer or other serious illness. No doctor, no macrobiotic counselor, no family member can do this for you.

In Conclusion

It is clear that modern medicine has been unsuccessful in its attempts to control cancer. Yet the diagnosis of cancer need not be accepted with despair and resignation. Through lifestyle change and a process of really getting in touch with yourself, you can become one of those people who says, "Thank God I had cancer, it has changed my whole life!" Patricia Reis, our therapist at Women to Women, summarizes this beautifully: "The bigger meaning of healing is a wholeing, a filling out of the missing pieces of a person's life. Sometimes this may mean coming to face death in a more fully realized way. Certainly it is an opportunity to come more deeply and fully into life."

References

Bailar and Smith, "Progress Against Cancer," *New England Journal of Medicine*, May 8, 1986, pp. 1226–1232.

Cairns, John, "The Treatment of Diseases and The War Against Cancer," *Scientific American*, November 1985, Vol. 253, No. 5, pp. 51–59

Maran, Meredith, "After Cancer, The Problems of Surviving," *Medical Self Care*, May–June 1986

Schaef, Anne Wilson, *When Society Becomes An Addict*, Harper & Row, 1987

Resources

- Exceptional Cancer Patients
  2 Church Street South

New Haven, CT 06519
(203) 865–8392
Sponsors workshops and lectures on optimizing healing potential. Based on the work of Bernie Siegal, M.D. List of audio and video tapes available.

- American Holistic Medical Foundation/Association
2727 Fairview Avenue East
Seattle, WA 98102
(206) 322–6842
Newsletter, publications and research in holistic medicine. Sponsors conferences. Referral source for holistic health care practitioners.

- Grobstein, Clifford, *Diet, Nutrition and Cancer*, 1982
National Academy Press
2101 Constitution Avenue NW
Washington D. C. 20418
Authoritative review of the role of diet in cancer prevention and treatment.

- Siegal, Bernie, *Love, Medicine and Miracles*, Harper & Row, 1986

- "Fight For Your Life: Survival Techniques For Those With Cancer."
This excellent video presentation was developed especially for cancer patients. It contains several techniques and exercises that can be used every day to help fight against cancer; four cancer survivors and Bernie Siegal, M.D. are interviewed. "It teaches how to become a survivor and live to tell your story, too."
Order from Varied Directions. Call 1–800–225–5669 toll-free.

Stress, Nutrition, and Immunity: Toward a Harmony of Self

Martha C. Cottrell, M.D. with Mark Mead

The Conventional View of Stress

Keeping well is usually described as care of the body through proper nutrition and exercise, avoidance of alcohol and tobacco, immunization against disease and adequate medical care when needed. This approach, however, while entirely valid, is not complete. A growing body of scientific evidence has shown that psychological and nutritional factors can *collectively* either cause disease or modulate the expression of disease caused by other factors, such as dietary carcinogens, industrial chemicals, viral infections, bacterial toxins, and allergens. Understanding of mind-body dynamics within the human organism, together with nutritional and psychosocial influences, may help reorient the health-care industry away from the prevailing emphasis on disease correction toward a greater emphasis on health promotion and maintenance. The study of stress and its relationship to well-being is surely a fundamental step in this more enlightened direction.

Books and articles on stress-related problems have traditionally emphasized symptoms of stress—high blood pressure, erratic emotional states, headaches, muscle cramping and tension. The approaches suggested to combat stress include meditation, relaxation, yoga, massage, biofeedback, tranquilizers, psychiatric assistance, and simply "learning to cope with stress." Workshops on stress management have asserted that if people become aware that the stress they are under is limiting their performance or life experience, they can overcome the identified stresses through sheer effort. A similar theme is echoed in Dr. Herbert Benson's *The Relaxation Response* and other popular books which advocate specific techniques for reducing blood pressure and alleviating the symptoms of stress.

These theories have merit, but by and large they seem limited and short-sighted. The basis for this criticism is essentially three-fold:

First, these approaches seek out symptoms rather than causes. The orientation is analogous to someone who stops his car when the red oil light goes on but, rather than putting in more oil, snips the wires connected to the oil light. Techniques to reduce the effects of stress are only remedial and at best a temporary solution. Logic, common sense, and experience tell us that the way to prevent and relieve the symptoms of distress is first to understand the role of our perception of stress, next to learn to identify those stressors (agents which provoke an adaptive response) which are changeable or controllable, and finally to discern those which are unchangeable but to which we can adapt through an appropriate change in perspective. An integrated understanding of these basic elements is essential in getting to the true roots of stress and stress-related problems.

Second, drug-oriented and psychiatric approaches have generally dealt with the individual as an object to be categorized, analyzed, manipulated, and sedated. This leaves the power of one's own ability or will to heal out of the picture. Our understanding of the highly individualized nature of susceptibility to stress, together with body-mind interrelationships, makes it imperative that people feel truly capable of healing themselves. A sound approach should be designed to instill this sense of personal autonomy and empowerment. Once such an attitude is established within the individual and his own will enters the process, the appropriate response to stress and the ability to establish disease resistance becomes consistent and integrated into his lifestyle.

Third, there is a need for greater emphasis on environmental and psychosocial factors operating at a deeper, more subtle level. These factors are reflected in the broad spectrum of environmental and psychosocial changes that have dramatically impacted modern civilization over the course of this century. History shows that the human body has a great capacity to adapt and thrive in its natural environment and to effectively attend to its own needs. Over millions of years of evolution, Homo sapiens has survived the ravages of sudden climatic change, attacks of wild animals, and various extremes in living conditions. And yet, although our ancestors had a tremendous capacity to adapt, their quality of life and the nature of their stress was vastly different from our own.

Furthermore our research indicates that, while stress has always been with us and will continue to be with us, the current plethora of stress-related symptoms is of relatively recent origin. Logically, we may look to major changes in living conditions that have taken place over the last 150 years and particularly since the early part of this century. A few of the most radical changes are rising economic pressures and material expectations, increasing toxicity in the environment, and a marked reduction in the quality of nutrition. These are important underlying sources of stress for which we have varying degrees of control. Since the role of nutrition has been almost entirely overlooked in stress management, it will be considered here for its dual role as both a stressor and as a vital support for one's response to stress.

In order to go beyond the conventional view of stress as a fragmented phenomenon (mind *or* body as opposed to mind *and* body), our perspective strives to integrate the fundamental relationships between: (a) mind and immunity, (b) nutrition and immunity, and (c) nutrition and mind. It is also acknowledged that patterns of social conditioning have influenced many of our belief systems and habitual behaviors, for example, that having a cup of coffee and a cigarette is an effective way to handle stress, when in fact the effects of nicotine and caffeine compound the stress in a cumulative manner. In short, no one factor alone is more important than any other, though some, such as dietary practices, affect us in a more enduring way and are more within the realm of control than others.

Stress: Friend or Foe?

What do we mean by "stress," and what is its relationship to health and disease? To understand, let us first look at some basic aspects of the human body's functions. The body is made up of a highly intricate array of chemical substances which change constantly while carrying out diverse tasks such as movement, digestion, excretion, respiration and detoxification. The myriad changes must be kept within certain physiological bounds, however; blood pressure, heart rate, oxygen concentrations, and foodstuffs in the blood are constantly shifting to meet the demands of life. If any of these internal balancing mechanisms of *homeostasis* are altered too much, illness or premature death results. Disease itself may be seen as a condition in which bodily changes go beyond these limits, though not to the absolute limit the body can tolerate—which would result in death. Such homeostatic disturbances render the individual susceptible to outside agents such as viral and bacterial infections, malignancies and other forms of illness, and creates a tendency toward accidents, emotional disturbances, and so forth.

Some kinds of stress are controllable while others are noncontrollable. Controllable stresses might include dietary factors, thought patterns, job choice, and a plethora of mundane choices (whether to get a comfortable chair or car, etc.). Noncontrollable stress factors might include death of a loved one, economic recession, natural disasters, or acts of crime against ourselves. In addition, the capacity to respond appropriately or beneficially to stress is individualized, and depends on one's worldview, circumstances, and overall biological health. In other words, what may be stressful to one person may not affect another. "One man's pleasure is another man's pain."

Clearly, stress must be attended to at its source—we must learn to recognize and interpret controllable stresses. Furthermore, we must take steps to reinforce our biological adaptive responsiveness to stress—both controllable and noncontrollable—through proper nutrition and other aspects of a health-promoting lifestyle. Any other approach merely attempts to mask the symptoms or results of stress. By developing the means to reduce the total burden of stress upon the body, the intensity of the stress response will be lessened and the long-term effects will also be reduced.

Controllable factors which may contribute to disturbances in physiological balance include nutritional imbalances, coffee, alcohol, prescription drugs, antibiotics, food additives and toxic chemicals circulating in our air and water. They also include psychosocial influences such as poor self-esteem, repressed anger and hostility, unrealistic expectations and other distorted perceptions of self and society. Generally speaking, the body responds with rapid adjustments whenever any change threatens to go beyond the normal equilibrium parameters. Minor responses are effected collectively as an adaptive mechanism that enables us to go on living without "dis-ease," at least for the time being. We are here primarily concerned, however, with those conditions stated above which tend to bring about an inappropriate and detrimental response to stress.

Although stress is usually spoken of as harmful, it is in fact normal and even essential, serving to maintain us throughout our daily life events and circumstances. Recent research has shown that several glands and organs play important roles in the body's response to stress. Hans Seyle, M.D., a long-standing authority on the study of stress, has emphasized the role of the adrenal glands. Among their most important functions, the adrenals secrete substances which regulate the distribution of body fluids and their dissolved mineral salts (hence playing a prominent role in maintaining proper blood pressure); releasing and building up stores of energy-supplying sugars; helping the body cope with infection; and allowing many other hormones and substances to work more effectively and safely throughout the body. Closely allied with adrenal functions are those of the immune and nervous systems. The changes induced by stress stimuli via the adrenals and nervous system mobilize the body's versatile immune mechanisms and reduce the possibilities of biologic breakdown, infection and degenerative disease.

Whether stress is supportive or non-supportive depends on the body's reaction to the stressor. Rather than being weakened, our resistance to disease may be bolstered by the stress of daily life; the stress response can raise the level of resistance to the stressor. For example, infection by viruses or bacteria elicits a rise in the manufacture of additional white blood cells and other immune components, which in turn eliminate the infectious agents. If the stress persists over time and becomes intensified, however, the mechanisms of immunity can become exhausted. At this point the individual "maladapts" to stress and succumbs to the throes of the disease process.

The body's biological reserves for responding to stress are not unlimited. Each bodily tissue or group of cells may be considered a miniature bank account in which money is deposited and utilized in the form of nutrients—proteins, fats, carbohydrates, vitamins and minerals. When spending is high, more money must be brought in to balance the budget. In like manner, when enzymes, hormones, antibodies, and other essential physiological components are called upon in some type of stress response, they must be rapidly replenished, and this ultimately depends on one's nutritional status. Nutrition thus serves invaluably by helping the body maintain sufficient reserves of immune components when presented with potentially adverse challenges or stresses. Furthermore, nutrition may indirectly alter immunity by influencing an individual's emotional temperament. This idea will be considered in more depth in a moment.

In sum, stress only becomes distress when our ability to respond appropriately to the stress stimuli is lacking or diminished. While stressors may be ubiquitous and inevitable—particularly in busy urban settings—the condition of *distress* is fundamentally our choice, a natural consequence of the way we think and conduct our daily lives. The key to effective stress management is having the mental clarity and energy, as well as the physiological adaptability, to deal with all varieties of stress.

An Emerging Medical Paradigm

There is now considerable evidence that the psychological effects of inappropriate modes of thought—stress, anxiety, mental tension—do not stay in the psyche. Rather, they are translated into the body where they eventuate in the symptoms of physical illness. Mind and body must therefore be considered as dynamically interconnected. By extension, virtually every physical disease has a psychosomatic component. Anger, loneliness, hopelessness, and low self-esteem—all based on habitual ways of thinking and of perceiving the world—have been associated with cancers, arthritis, diabetes, obesity, hypertension, and other degenerative diseases.[1] This biopsychosocial model posits that emotions and mental states can have an essential influence on the physiological functioning and infrastructure of an individual—a fact supported by substantial research in the rapidly expanding field of psycho-neuroimmunology.[2] For example, scientists have found that the brain can exercise direct control over cells of the immune system, that the two hemispheres of the brain influence immune function in different ways, and that certain brain chemicals (*neurotransmitters*), which ultimately depend upon nutritional status, have specific effects on immune competence.[3]

A key concept of stress research is that the nervous, hormonal, and immune systems are all intimately linked. We may take this a step further by viewing the integral influence of nutrition on all these systems, and hence on our overall responsiveness to stress. Nutrition provides the necessary extra support when bodily systems are confronted with additional sources of stress. The biologic relationships between nutritional factors, immunity, and brain function are extremely complex and beyond the scope of this article. The interested reader is urged to explore the list of references in the bibliography.[4,5]

As Fig. 1 indicates, there are two distinct biological causes of disease—heredity and environment. Hereditary predispositions include inherited weaknesses in certain body tissues or organs that increase susceptibility to disease. Environmental factors include viruses and bacteria, chemical toxins or pollutants, and dietary imbalances. A third integral cause is behaviorial. States of mind and emotional tendencies can sometimes determine whether processes that are initiated by hereditary or environmental factors will precipitate disease. In some cases, for example, psychological reactions appear to be precursors to intestinal malfunction and headache. These problems may have a concomitant organic cause in the form of chemical *allergens* (substances which trigger allergic reactions), or of nutritional imbalances or deficits, as will be outlined in a moment.

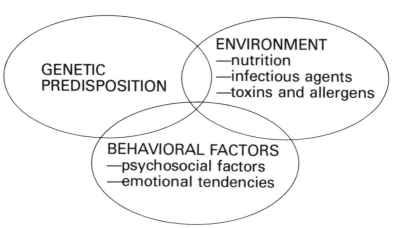

Fig. 1.   The Biopsychosocial Model of Health and Disease
The Biopsychosocial Model of Health and Disease, involving hereditary, environmental and behavioral factors in disease susceptibility.
By this view, disease can be caused by any of three variables acting
in conjunction. For example, some diseases implicate genetic factors,
while others seem to emphasize exposure to environmental agents like
artificial food additives and toxin-producing bacteria. Behavioral
variables or psychological states may interact by compromising
immune function, predisposing to infection, and increasing the likelihood of disease expression. Behavioral factors are closely aligned with
nutritional factors since dietary practice is voluntary and controllable.

Resolving Stress Naturally

The goal of stress management is twofold: (1) to create within
the individual a condition which promotes a relaxed yet alert
state of mind capable of concentration and clear thinking; and
(2) to establish a strong biological foundation capable of maximum resistance to stress. Optimum creativity and productivity
are a result of sound mental abilities and physical vitality, as
well as of course training and experience. Consider the issue of
time management in the office setting. Avoidance of interrup-
tions, proper scheduling, and delegation of authority is one way
to deal with management of time. But this problem can also be

dealt with at a deeper, "inside" level by addressing the physical and mental health of working individuals. Mental fatigue, confusion, and clouded thinking reflect one's physiological condition; as symptoms of declining health, they may also alter one's perception of time, consequently bringing about diminished productivity, creativity and success.

By and large, the various methods of meditation, visualization, self-hypnosis, relaxation techniques, yoga, tai-chi and other mind-body disciplines, have proven effective in altering our thoughts, attitudes and beliefs in a positive way. Added to these activities are various simple aspects of lifestyle such as taking a leisurely walk, immersing oneself in a creative hobby, breathing deeply, singing a song and having a good laugh. Finally, dietary practice fits into the picture by affecting both mind and body at the organic level. The role of diet in promoting health has received much attention by medical science over the past ten years; however, links between inappropriate nutritional status and degenerative conditions, both physical and mental, are highly varied and complex. Although the study of human dietary practices and biochemistry as they relate to stress is too complex to be covered in these pages, a few concepts are worth delving into here:

• *Excessive intake of simple sugars.*   One of the essential homeostatic balances in the body is the level of blood sugar, or *glucose*, which provides fuel to meet the body's energy needs. Whereas other body tissues can survive on amino acids and byproducts of fat digestion, the brain is utterly dependent upon glucose for its functioning. If blood sugar levels are normal, the body functions smoothly and the brain operates as both the central control panel and the organizer for rational human thought and behavior. However, any deficit of blood glucose results in an internal stress situation. Low blood sugar levels (*hypoglycemia*) have an acute effect on brain functions. Low blood sugar elicits a shutting down of biologically less essential brain functions to conserve the more essential, mechanical functions. The less essential area is the *cerebellum*, which controls the higher levels of human behavior, including love, hate, compassion, humor, and reasoning ability. When this occurs, one tends to revert to irrational behavioral tendencies governed by the *cerebrum*, which regulates breathing, heart action, and muscular activity in the "fight-or-flight" category (the panic response). Common symptoms of low blood sugar can include any of the following: insomnia and irregular sleep patterns; persistent tension headaches; compulsive sweet cravings; "shaky" or unsteady temperament; and extreme swings in mood. Also, when energy for the *cerebral cortex* (the area dealing with intellectual activity) is lacking due to low blood sugar, one experiences "brain fag" and a diminished ability to deal with challenging situations or to make critical split-second decisions. This results in a constant feeling of depression, anxiety, neurosis or other personality changes.

The primary causes of low blood sugar are diets high in sucrose or simple sugars (honey, tropical fruits, ice cream, candies, pastries and other white flour products), and low in fiber and complex carbohydrates. These foods cause extreme swings in the blood sugar level, going from very high to abnormally low. People often will take a cup of coffee or some other stimulant to pull them out of the energy lows of hypoglycemia. But this only compounds the problem further. To prevent and relieve low blood sugar, it is advisable to consume fiber-rich whole grains and vegetables, since these tend to produce a more sustained and gradual utilization of carbohydrate to meet the body's overall energy needs most efficiently.[5] The high-fiber content also helps detoxify the body by keeping fecal matter moving regularly through the intestines; any stagnation of intestinal function due to a slow-moving, fiber-deficient stool can result in gradual toxicity and a tendency toward hemorrhoids, diverticulosis, duodenal ulcer, gallstones, colon cancer and other cancers.[6]

• *Excessive intake of fats.* Diets high in fat tend to produce a clumping or sticking together of red blood cells (RBCs) in the bloodstream, leading to the RBCs' diminished capacity to bind and transport oxygen to the trillions of cells throughout the body, including the brain cells. This effect is amplified by clogging of the arteries due to fatty plaque build-up, a known contributor to hypertension and heart disease. Again, when organ tissues are inhibited from receiving oxygen and foodstuffs normally present in the bloodstream, they fail to function optimally and eventually degenerate. Deterioration of the brain, kidneys, adrenals and liver would seriously impair our ability to respond appropriately to stress. Reduction in blood flow due to high-fat diets may bring on prolonged fatigue, decreased endurance, and decreased work performance.[7,8] Improper breathing and inadequate exercise would further compound the problem. An additional concern is that toxic chemicals tend to concentrate in dietary fats and subsequently move to body fat, perhaps to eventually initiate disease processes.

Fats, or fatty acids, are integral components of all cell membranes, and can influence the flow of substances (nutrients, ions, enzymes, etc.) in and out of cells. A high saturated-fat content in the membrane may adversely alter the physical structure and electrical charge of the immunologic receptors on cells, resulting in abnormal recognition of viruses, bacteria, or other antigens.[9] It is important to note, however, that *any* excess of dietary fats, whether saturated or unsaturated (including so-called *essential fatty acids*), can have undesirable consequences and weaken one's overall immunocompetence.[10] This includes altered functioning of antibodies and various key immune cells.[11] Diets that generally minimize fat entirely are the best choice. This again brings out the efficacy of consuming a diet of cereal grains, vegetables, beans, fruits, nuts and seeds.

• *Excessive intake of protein.* Regular consumption of red meats, eggs, cheese, milk, poultry, and fish may lead to various imbalances in the body, including deterioration of kidney function through the excessive production of *uric acids*, a metabolic byproduct of protein digestion. Uric acids, sulfates, and other acidic byproducts of high-protein consumption are toxic to the body's tissues and constitute a major internal stressor. The body is constantly striving to maintain a slightly alkaline blood condition. When there is temporary acidity, one experiences fatigue and lethargy, and a general weakening of physiological functions occurs.

Heavy consumption of protein also has a direct adverse effect on brain chemistry. The brain produces *serotonin*, a neurotransmitter that has a calming effect in times of stress. *Tryptophan*, an amino acid used by the brain to make serotonin, can be found in high concentrations in most animal products and legumes. The ability of serotonin-containing neurons to synthesize serotonin depends on the level of tryptophan in the brain, which in turn is ultimately determined by our daily diet. However, the extra amounts of amino acids released from high-protein digestion compete with tryptophan transport, thereby restricting the brain's ability to utilize tryptophan.[12] By contrast, through a mechanism involving insulin secretion, high-carbohydrate meals *elevate* brain tryptophan and serotonin concentration.[13] Complex carboydrate-rich, low-protein foods such as grains and vegetables, promote more efficient uptake of tryptophan for the production of serotonin and *endorphins* (multi-functional compounds involved in the alleviation of anxiety and pain, as well as the stimulation of immune function).

Recent research shows that other dietary substances act on the two complementary parts of the involuntary (autonomic) nervous system, the sympathetic and parasympathetic systems. The *sympathetic nervous system* (which controls adrenal output and the "fight-or-flight" stress response) is balanced by the *parasympathetic system* (which regulates secretion, glandular activity, blood flow, and general maintenance). Excessive parasympathetic activity has been correlated with depressive states, whereas sympathetic excesses are correlated with states of anxiety.[14] Two chemical substances, *choline* and *tyrosine*, function as neurotransmitter precursors to affect the parasympathetic and sympathetic responses to stress. The major physiological chemical influencing parasympathetic functions is called *acetycholine* and is directly proportional to the amount of choline in our diet. Eggs and meats are the richest sources of choline. By stimulating the parasympathetic system, acetycholine can induce increased stomach acid secretion, excessive bowel action and glandular responses which relate to feelings of anger and frustration.[15] Diets low in choline may thereby tend to bring on a more relaxed state, with decreased aggressive drives and a more contemplative mood. The other substance, tyrosine, is also found in high concentrations in red meats and dairy products, particularly aged cheese. Tyrosine supports the production of the thyroid hormone, *thyroxine*, which tends to increase the activity of the sympathetic nervous system such as adrenalin secretion. Hyperalert states, anxiety and poor digestion, may all result from high tyrosine ingestion.[16]

Protein can be appropriately obtained by regularly consuming whole cereal grains, beans, and nuts and seeds, as well as small quantities of fish and seafood two or more times per week. For the reasons stated above and for those voiced elsewhere, red meats, eggs, and dairy products should generally be avoided or minimized. As illustrated in Frances Moore Lappe's *Diet for a Small Planet*, protein needs may be readily met by adhering to a strict and well-rounded vegetarian diet.

• *Food additives.* The category of food additives includes all pre-servatives, coloring agents, flavoring enhancers, texturizers, and fragrances, as well as agricultural chemicals—pesticides, herbi-cides, and fungicides. According to Samuel Epstein in *The Politics of Cancer*, the average American eats nine pounds of chemical additives a year. Longterm consumption of food additives may result in birth defects, organ damage, and cancer.[17] Nitrites and nitrates, used as preservatives in packaged meats and found in a variety of animal products, are converted to nitrosamines, which appear to be associated with stomach and other gastrointestinal cancers.[18] Artificial sweeteners such as saccharin and cyclamate have been linked with the development of bladder cancer.[19]

Although it is difficult to know the full range of long-term effects of the three thousand or more chemicals that have in-filtrated our food supply, recent data suggests that they are doing more harm than good. The immune and detoxification mechanisms of the body must labor much harder when confronted with these substances, and this drains energy that could be used for bodily homeostatic processes on the micro level, and for constructive work and solid play on the macro level. In addition, many of these toxic substances weaken organs important in the body's adap-tability to common types of stress. A diet virtually free of addi-tives is an essential first step in establishing sound immunity and biological functioning overall, and organically grown grains and vegetables are by far the best alternative. Recall also that even conventionally farmed plant foods tend to concentrate less chemicals than do animal products.

• *Vitamin and mineral imbalances.* The importance of procurring vitamins and minerals in the form of an unrefined and nonfortified grain-and-vegetable-based diet cannot be overemphasized. The differences in the physiological and biochemical effects of consuming supplements versus whole foods are considerable. For this reason the National Academy of Sciences, in their 1982 landmark publication, *Diet, Nutrition and Cancer*, stated that nutrition from whole foods is far more preferable than from vitamin and mineral supplements. (The thirteen-member scientific committee also recommended reducing substantially the consumption of foods high in saturated and unsaturated fat and increasing the daily intake of whole grains, vegetables, and fruit.[20]) Keep this in mind when considering the following body of evidence for the health benefits of single nutrients. The goal is to see how all are dynamically interwoven as integral parts of the whole.

Below is a small sampling of the findings on the relationship between micronutrient balance and immune competence:

Vitamins

(1) **Vitamin A**, or *retinol*, has for many years been recognized for its role in *nonspecific* resistance to infectious disease by helping to preserve the integrity of skin and mucous membranes, the protective barriers against infectious microorganisms. The vitamin is also needed for the production of anti-bacterial lysozymes in tears, saliva, and sweat.[21] In terms of *specific* immunity, diets deficient in vitamin A have resulted in significantly depressed antibody production and other immune responses.[22,23,24,25] Vitamin A has been shown to enhance the activity of immune cells against tumor cells.[26,27,28] The functioning of key regulatory immune cells is also enhanced by vitamin A levels, and this may constitute an important aspect of the anticancer action of retinoids.[29] Vitamin A also works as an *antioxidant* to protect the integrity of cells against harmful elements in the environment, and this is thought to play a key role in protection against cancer.[30]

Dietary Sources: Vitamin A is procurred primarily in the form of the provitamin, *beta carotene*, which forms part of the pigments of many green and yellow vegetables. Excellent sources include: carrots, collard greens, kohlrabi, kale, broccoli, parsley, turnip greens, dandelion greens, mustard greens, watercress, leek greens, endive, chicory, pumpkin, and squash (acorn, butternut, and hubbard). Sea vegetables and various forms of freshwater algae are also high in beta carotene.

2) **B-Complex Vitamins** are comprised of a group of substances usually found grouped together in nature. Some of the more prominent of the B-complex vitamins are pyridoxine, colbalamin, thiamin, riboflavin, niacin, folic acid, and pantothenic acid. Vitamin B_6, or *pyridoxine*, participates crucially in the direct line of protein, carbohydrate and lipid metabolism, and acts as a coenzyme consituent in amino acid metabolism and in red blood cell formation.[31] Pyridoxine has demonstrated the ability to inhibit tumor growth.[32] A deficiency of this vitamin depresses both cellular and humoral immunity.[33] For instance, diminished antibody production is observed following stimulation by foreign substances (*antigens*),[34] and immune cells exhibit abnormal proliferation when stimulated by antigens.[35] Pantothenic acid deficiency and folic acid deficiency are each associated with decreases in lymphatic organ size, immune cell ratios, spleen cell response, serum antibody levels, primary and secondary antibody responses, and resistance to infection.[36] There is also decreased immune inhibition of tumor growth.[37] Pantothenic acid deficiency appears to inhibit the stimulation of antibody-producing cells and their ability to produce new antibodies.[38] Thiamin and riboflavin are milder immunity promoters which, under deficiency conditions, generally elicit the same set of immunological effects listed above. As with the other B vitamins, they play a key role in such physiological functions as maintenance of mucosal membranes, formation of red blood cells, and metabolism of carbohydrates.

Dietary Sources: Preferable sources for these B vitamins include brown rice, wheat, barley, oats, corn, rye, soybean and soy products (*miso*, *tempeh*, *tamari*, and *tofu*), kidney, and other

beans, broccoli, Brussels sprouts, kale, kohlrabi, turnips, cabbage
endive, parsely, parsnips, dandelion greens, watercress, cauli
flower, lentils, leeks, almonds, walnuts, peanuts and chicory, anc
various species of white-meat fish (cod, flounder, etc.).[39]

Vitamin B_{12} (*cobalamin*) may exert an important influence or
key regulatory cells of the immune system called *T-helper* anc
T-suppressor cells.[40] A deficiency leads to a wide variety of diminished immune functions.[41] Vitamin B_{12} participates along witl
folic acid in the synthesis of the hemoglobin in red blood cells
and contributes to cell longevity, DNA and RNA synthesis, whit
blood cell longevity, health of the central nervous system, anc
metabolism of carbohydrates, fats, and proteins.[42]

Dietary Sources: Foods providing B_{12} in the standard macro
biotic diet are miso, tempeh, *natto*, tamari, sea vegetables, pickles
fish and some unwashed organically grown vegetables. Vitamir
B_{12} is required in extremely small amounts—less than one milliontl
of a gram (1 mcg). This vitamin can be obtained in sufficien
quantity in macrobiotic diets if one gives proper attention tc
food selection and preparation, to the way of eating, and to othei
aspects of lifestyle such as physical activity. For instance, one
should ' guard against overcooking and excessive washing o'
organic produce, since these practices tend to eliminate B_{12}-pro
ducing bacteria harbored in these foods.

(3)   **Vitamin C**, or *ascorbic acid*, seems to play a role in sup
porting overall immune functioning. Humans and animals fec
ascorbic acid-deficient diets are more susceptible to infectiou
diseases that controls fed adequate vitamin C diets, and hav
reduced levels of both humoral and cell-mediated responses.[4]
Vitamin C essentially supports *phagocyte* (cells which consume
toxic debris and potential pathogens) migration and functioning
as well as the healing of wounds.[44] It may also influence immunity
indirectly by boosting one's psychoneurologic capacity to dea
with stress: it counteracts the immunosuppressive effects of *corti
costeroids* (natural stress-induced hormones), yet simultaneousl
assists in the anti-inflammatory function of the steroids.[45] Ascorbi

acid also acts as an antioxidant and free-radical scavenger and thus may protect against cancer by preventing the formation of carcinogens and tumors in the body (e.g., inhibits the formation of carcinogenic nitrosamines from nitrites—breakdown byproducts of most barbequed meats—by reacting with the nitrites).[46,47] Note also that it has a synergistic effect when taken with other antioxidants, that is to say, the more vitamin C one takes, the less vitamin E one needs, and visa versa.[48]

Dietary Sources: Superb sources include broccoli, Brussels sprouts, collards, kale, parsley, turnip greens, carrot tops, sprouts, cabbage, cauliflower, kohlrabi, mustard greens, watercress, and strawberries (for dessert, of course). Also, because cooking may easily cause loss of this vitamin, gentle steaming is preferable to boiling or heavy steaming.

(4) **Vitamin E**: This vitamin aids in the formation of red blood cells (RBCs), and helps maintain the integrity of the vascular and central nervous systems, as well as the kidney tubules, lungs, genitals, liver, and RBC membranes. In animal studies, diets supplemented with vitamin E led to an enhanced antibody production when challenged by infectious microorganisms.[49] Elevated vitamin E levels in the blood, in addition to raising the antibody response, have been observed to improve white cell bactericidal activity and phagocytosis.[50] A deficiency in vitamin E has been shown to result in decreased lymphatic organ size, immune cell proliferation, white blood cell function, inflammatory response, and host resistance to infection.[51] Also, the antioxidant properties of this vitamin protect the lungs from air pollution damage. During stress there are increased requirements of cortisone and vitamin E, and there is a high content of vitamin E at sites of cortisone synthesis in the adrenal glands.[52]

Dietary Sources: The best dietary sources for this vitamin are the following: whole wheat berries, barley, brown rice, oats, rye, corn and sesame oils, miso, tofu, tempeh, natto, sesame and alfalfa seeds, dark leafy greens, and lightly roasted nuts such as walnuts, almonds, and peanuts.

Next let us consider the essential roles of minerals, which are somewhat arbitrarily divided into two categories: major minerals, or bulk elements, and trace elements. The major minerals include calcium, phosphorous, iodine, sulfur, magnesium, sodium, and potassium. The trace elements include cadmium, chromium, cobalt, copper, iron, manganese, molybdenum, selenium, and zinc. Minerals function as essential enzyme cofactors in metabolic reactions; as components of organic compounds (e.g., in enzymes, hormones, and other compounds); as ions affecting muscle contractility; and as minerals in bone structure. Every chemical process in the body requires minerals of varying kinds and proportions.

(1) **Zinc:** Zinc is required for normal growth and development and plays an integral part in numerous metabolic processes. It is also a necessary ingredient in T-cell functioning, which provides immunity against infectious organisms and tumor development. A deficiency can produce atrophy of the thymus gland and a reduction in the number of mature T cells. As a result, many cell-mediated immune functions are impaired, including T- and B-cell bactericidal activity, natural-killer-cell activity, and other immune responses.[53] Low levels of zinc have been associated with reduced antibody response, abnormal proportions of antibodies, and defective cell-mediated immunity.[54] Patients with immunodeficiency diseases, in addition to the typical array of depressed immune responses, frequently exhibit low levels of serum zinc; and repletion is associated with the restoration of many of these immune functions.[55] It is also interesting that a hallmark of the physiological response to invasion by pathogenic microorganisms or their toxins is a transient decline in serum zinc, with a concomitant sequestering of zinc from the liver.[56]

Dietary Sources: Prominent dietary sources for zinc include cooked whole wheat, brown rice, rye, barley, oats, buckwheat, oysters, tuna, shrimp, crab, sunflower and pumpkin seeds, various sea vegetables (*kombu, wakame,* etc.), corn, lentils, peas, watercress, parsley, okra, and carrots.

(2) **Manganese**: Manganese appears to be important in the maintenance of structural integrity of heart and kidney cell membranes, tissue oxygen uptake, food absorption, neurotransmitter synthesis (affecting brain function and cerebral activity), fertility, insulin synthesis, fat carbohydrate metabolism, and homeostatic blood-clotting mechanisms.[57] It is a component of an antioxidant called *superoxide dismutase*, and there is some evidence that it may help to counteract the immunosuppressive effects of corticosteroids.[58] Although much is known about the immunosuppressive effects of excess manganese, relatively little is known about its specific positive effects on the immune system. The most likely effects would be on the plasma membranes of important cell types employed in the immune response, since changes in membrane structure of fluidity could in turn influence the binding affinity for antibodies and immune cells.[59] At this point it seems likely that manganese influences immunocompetence predominantly by indirect means, for example, as a key component of carbohydrate and lipid metabolism, as an antioxidant, and as a cofactor in various enzyme systems.

Dietary Sources: The most abundant and balanced sources of manganese are the following: cooked brown rice, barley, oats, buckwheat, rye, whole wheat, kelp, wakame, kombu, dulse, sunflower seeds, almonds, walnuts, parsley, celery, Brussel sprouts, broccoli, watercress, kale and other dark leafy greens. Spinach is high in manganese but contains *oxalic acid*, which renders the mineral largely unavailable.

(3) **Copper**: Copper plays an essential role in respiration, and functions as a cofactor for many important enzymes, called *cuproenzymes*, which catalyze oxidation reactions. By and large, however, copper's most significant role is as an integral structural feature of many enzymes in metabolic processes. Deficiency of this element has been linked to lowered resistance to infectious challenge[60] and shortened lifespan and greatly increased mortality following infection.[61] Copper appears to be essential to proper functioning of a wide range of cell types, including antibody-forming cells, T helper cells, macrophages, and certain types of white blood cells.[62] Both dietary excess and dietary deficiency

can have negative effects on these cell populations. The trace element also seems to be involved in the inflammatory process, at certain times potentiating and at certain times inhibiting it.[63] Finally, copper is intimately involved in the three-dimensional structure of antibodies.[64]

Dietary Sources: Favorable sources of dietary copper include the following: cooked whole wheat, barley, oats, rye, rice, almonds, walnuts, sunflower and sesame seeds, miso, tofu, tempeh, natto, kale, onions, leeks, okra, sea vegetables, and various species of non-fatty, white-meat fish. Zinc and copper have a delicate inverse interrelationship in the body and tend to interact antagonistically to one another. Because of the extremely narrow range of our copper needs, zinc supplementation may elicit copper deficiency, and too much copper may upset the zinc balance.

Additional Concerns
Regarding Micronutrient Balance

It is of particular concern that the average American diet, which is high in animal products and refined sugars, may be lacking in several of the important micronutrients, both marginally and proportionately. Such trace element and vitamin imbalances could, in turn, alter the functional integrity of the immune and nervous systems. It should be noted that many of our present foodcrops are deficient in certain essential trace elements (e.g., selenium, manganese, copper, and zinc) and minerals (e.g., iron and magnesium) as a result of conventional farming practices.[65,66] The use of soluble fertilizers—artificial preparations of predominantly nitrates, phosphates, and potash—causes imbalances in the soil mineral composition, and trace elements are gradually washed away along with the soil's valuable humus content. Mineral-deficient soils then produce mineral-deficient plant foods. Animal products, too, are deficient, since domestic animals depend on plant sources for food. Furthermore, the intensive cultivation and monoculture practices of conventional farming lead to soil erosion, the loss of valuable topsoil and a tragic gross loss of minerals altogether! Taken together, these points warrant further investigation of trace-mineral availability in the nation's food supply. If these micronutrients are truly lacking, then our immune systems stand a risk of becoming seriously compromised.

Beyond health-threatening agricultural practices, intensive food-processing in the American food system further contributes to the problem of micronutrient imbalance. Consider chromium, another of the essential trace elements, and particularly noted for its potential role in carbohydrate metabolism and in preventing diabetes and heart disease. Americans in general had extremely low levels of chromium when compared to subjects from other parts of the world. Oriental peoples averaged 4.5 times as much and other nationalities also had markedly more chromium in the blood.[67] Interestingly, compared to Western societies, Oriental populations tend to have markedly lower incidence of diabetes and heart disease, although their prevalence has been increasing rapidly since the 1950s in Japan and other areas of modernization.[68] Refined carbohydrate foods are extremely low in chromium since it is lost through refining processes. In grains, for example, chromium is contained in the outer bran portion, so much is lost in the production of white flour. In this case, there is also an additive effect since our body's chromium needs increase in proportion to blood carbohydrate levels; thus higher intakes of simple sugars per se tend to deplete the body of chromium.[69]

The average American diet also tends to lack in B-complex vitamins and in balanced proportions of these micronutrients. This, again, is largely a result of heavy reliance on refined cereal-grain products, sugary foods, and adulterated or highly processed foods in general. Excessive caloric intakes (overeating) may also contribute by upsetting the digestive system. In addition, metabolism of carbohydrates and proteins, when consumed in excess, requires a larger supply of various B vitamins. Note that some of these vitamins have an integral relationship with bacterial colonization in the large intestine, and this may have some bearing on antibiotics' capacity to alter the balance of B-complex vitamins in the body.[70] This is a nice example of how some of the finer physiological interrelationships of the body may indirectly influence immunocompetence.

Trace elements influence physiological, genetic, and psychological aspects of development from prenatal life through the stages of growth, maintenance, and aging.[71] Trace-element deficiencies are not peculiar to malnourished children of underdeveloped countries, but also manifest to an unknown extent in affluent or industrial countries.[72] For example, some observations suggest that marginal copper deficiency may occur widely throughout the population of the United States.[73] In light of the many studies suggesting an integral relationship between trace-element balance and the health of the nervous system, the possibility of borderline deficiencies or imbalances supporting learning disabilities, abnormal behavior and other psychological problems, offers grounds for concern.[74]

There has been some concern that mineral deficiencies may also result by consuming a high fiber, vegetarian diet. Earlier laboratory studies found that fiber binds minerals in the intestine and could therefore inhibit their absorption. This theory has recently been contradicted by a recent investigation which found no evidence of mineral deficiency for people on long-term, high-fiber vegetarian diets.[75] Oxalic acid binds minerals such as zinc, copper, iron and calcium and can inhibit their absorption. Since this acid is found in certain of the green vegetables, including green peppers, spinach, Swiss chard and tomatoes, it may be wise to avoid or minimize their use. These considerations are all part of the standard macrobiotic dietary approach.

Beyond Diet: the Realm of Awareness

The macrobiotic approach begins with the realization that the environment itself is orderly and supportive; and further, that human life is an integral part of this constantly changing, harmonious fabric. The central problem in establishing sound health lies in our way of thinking. The mind can create an illusory sense of dualism which emphasizes the antagonistic and neglects the complementary nature of things. For example, a hard-driving, work superior can often appear to be a monster—someone who causes you to "stress out"—but he or she is also likely to push you to greater performance and achievement. Seeing the front and back of every situation requires an acknowledgment that, as quantum physics has revealed, the universe is unified and orderly, not fragmented and chaotic. Falsely seeing oneself confronted by a world of separate existences, one creates in one's mind a reality of seemingly irreconcilable antagonisms, and this generally produces tension and anxiety. Awareness of an integrated, harmonious universe can provide a profoundly stable base for growing, rather than deteriorating, as a result of life's myriad stresses.

One of the most subtle and ubiquitous sources of stress in the modern world is our awareness of time. Time is commonly regarded as a linear reality consisting of past, present, and future— a conception based on three dimensional perception. However, as Einstein proposed in his Special Theory of Relativity, and as was later verified by quantum physics and Jungian depth psychology, the perception of linear time is an illusion. The notion that time flows in a one-way fashion is a property of consciousness. As Larry Dossey, M.D., states in his book, *Space, Time, and Medicine.* "The sensation of [linear, unidirectional] time flow belongs to the mind, and not to nature itself."[76] Units of time are mere practical constructs of rational thought which appear to give meaning to our daily existence.

Dossey makes a good case for the healing value of the "here and now" consciousness. Being absorbed in one's activity in each passing moment better enables one to relinquish fear (of future mishaps) and guilt (over past errors), and thereby opens one up to the possibilities of the present. Yet such an orientation requires keen focus and concentration, especially when confronted with a complex or psychologically demanding situation. Meditation, visualization, and various relaxation techniques can help one establish such a one-pointed mind. Furthermore, studies of the relationship between nutrition and mental health suggest that such consciousness can be supported biologically through diet. High sugar intake, lack of minerals, and excessive additives in the diet can alter one's ability to concentrate or think clearly and rationally. A grain-and-vegetable-based diet, by promoting sustained and regular energy levels, as well as minimizing toxicity to the human organism, is ideal biological support for the complex, integrated array of electrochemical activities which underlies the higher neurological functions of thought and behavior.

Through awareness of the value of being fully present, one comes to focus on the experience of each moment, and thus chooses those things which will continually enhance the quality of life. This, in turn, creates the opportunity for living, growing, and evolving toward the highest human achievement—the awareness of the connectedness of all things and the infinite order of life. In this state of awareness, one appreciates the natural order of things as observed and experienced through the cyclic movements of summer and winter, light and dark, birth and death, happiness and strife, acceptance and denial, wholeness and fragmentation, and so on. In acknowledging the truth of this perpetual flow of orderly change, and extending this sense of truth to our own lives, we are better able to appreciate personal events and experiences as necessary in our evolution toward greater wholeness. Acceptance of the rightness and fairness of natural order frees one from regret over past mistakes or fear of future tribulations, and can heighten one's ability to create harmony in daily life.

According to the macrobiotic perspective, illness is a manifestation of imbalance within the organism. Understanding the totality of this imbalance enables one to direct one's way of life toward the recovery of balance. Illness is not seen as a matter of chance, morality or divine punishment, but merely as a reflection of one's ignorance of natural order, and thus as an opportunity for learning, growth, and enlightenment. In particular, the experience of disease affords the possibility for expanding awareness of the relationship between self and the environment, which in turn underlies the responsibility for one's entire well-being. Such personal responsibility encompasses one's sense of empowerment and the ability to transform one's condition from sickness to health, or imbalance to balance. This view contrasts sharply with the common view of the individual as a victim of cruel fate (i.e., viruses, bacteria, fungi, etc.), a view which actually disempowers the individual and leaves him fearful, confused, and impotent.

The recognition that one is solely responsible for oneself and one's world does not mean that one has literally created the world, nor that the world is merely a figment of one's imagination. It means, rather, that the meaning of the world, its events, objects, and people, are all determined by one's mode of perception—one's own worldview or paradigm. If one feels discontent or unhappy, it is ultimately due to a distorted perception and dualistic interpretation of the situation at hand: one has assigned false or fragmentary meaning to the presumed "cause" of one's unhappiness. Changing one's negative emotional state may therefore entail two steps: (1) working through the emotional energy in a constructive way (meditation, movement, etc.); and (2) making a fundamental change in one's total perspective. It is this latter step to which macrobiotics makes its greatest contribution in the area of psychosocial problems. Macrobiotics offers us a profound perceptual tool for seeing the universe as a harmonious, orderly organism, operating for the benefit of all creatures within it. As Jesus said in *The Gospel According to Thomas*: "The Kingdom of Heaven is spread upon the earth, yet men do not see it."

Conclusion

Unless we recognize that we determine our health and happiness through our own patterns of daily living, we will never know true health. Once we assume some measure of mindful control over these influences, distress rapidly abates, energy and enthusiasm are encouraged, and creativity and joie de vivre naturally blossom forth. With sound health, exposures to stress can further strengthen one's overall condition and general resistance. One's capacity to cope with similar pressures, without developing an extreme stress reaction, will be enhanced when the practical measures outlined above are employed. In short, stress becomes our friend which makes us stronger and our life more enjoyable.

The Chinese word for crisis is written by combining the symbols for the words "danger" and "opportunity." This reflects the enlightened "front-and-back" awareness mentioned previously. Stress is both positive and negative—a danger and an opportunity, a friend and a foe. Taking responsibility for our bodies and minds by living in a more health-supporting way is the crux to actually realizing profound growth potential with which stress presents us.

Biomedical science could greatly enhance the effects of medical treatments and the approach to stress-related disorders by emphasizing the importance of nutrition, exercise, and lifestyle modification. Holistic practitioners, on the other hand, would enhance their position by recognizing the necessity, in some instances, of employing conventional (allopathic) technologies, especially in the area of acute crisis situations and "runaway" infectious conditions. *The key to reconciliation between orthodox and unorthodox approaches is in realizing the appropriateness of each with respect to the individual afflicted by illness.* Ultimately there may come a day when holistic and allopathic doctors work side by side, complementing the other's expertise and knowledge, and thus offering optimal health care.

Going further, psychobiological research has demonstrated profound and highly complex connections between nutrition and psychological states. Dietary balance and quality of mind thus lie on a continuum. Based on an integrated view of nutrition and psychoneuroimmunology, it seems logical that recovery from immunologic disease may be promoted by a combination of fundamental biochemical *and* psychological changes induced by adopting a grain-based diet *and* a comprehensive philosophy of life. The synergistic interaction of healthy body and harmonious emotions would greatly support the functioning of the immune system and may enhance recovery from even the most degenerative conditions. This possibility was amply born out by Dr. Anthony Sattilaro's dramatic recovery from "terminal" cancer, as portrayed in his superb book, *Recalled by Life.*

A comprehensive approach to health and disease requires balanced consideration of all factors: biological, psychosocial, environmental, and spiritual. The essential gift of the macrobiotic approach is in providing the practical means to accomplish this end. Furthermore, if we can avail ourselves to studying the macrobiotic perspective, we may gain valuable insights into recoveries that have heretofore been dismissed as "anecdotal," or looked upon as instances of "spontaneous remission" (in which ostensibly terminal cancer is halted and disappears). Medical science's labeling of "spontaneous" connotes a view of illness as a chance or capricious event, which in turn tacitly contradicts the view of illness as a logical process and manifestation of inner organic imbalances. This somewhat mystical attitude no longer serves us well and must ultimately give way to a more dynamic, ecological and integrated perspective founded on universal principles. If we can humbly acknowledge that we are still limited in our understanding of how disease develops, we may open ourselves to new possibilities for creating a healthier world.

"No mind can embrace a new idea until it rejects the alternatives."
—John Stuart Mill

References

[1] Pelletier, K. (1977) "Personality and emotions in cancer," in: *Mind as Healer, Mind as Slayer*. Delta Publishing Co., N.Y., N.Y. pp. 134–149

[2] Locke, S. E. and M. Hornig-Rohan (1983) *Mind and Immunity*: Behavioral Immunology, An Annotated Bibliography, 1976–1982. Institute for the Advancement of Health, 16 East 53rd St. N.Y., N.Y. 10022

[3] Schmeck, H. M. (1985) "By training the brain, scientists find links to immune defenses." *The New York Times*, Jan. 1., 1985

[4,5] Several superb medical texts on this subject include the following:

● Gershwin, M. E. et al. (1985) *Nutrition and Immunity*. Academic Press, Inc., N.Y.

● Chandra, R. K. (1980) *Immunology of Nutritional Disorders*. Year Book Medical Publishers, Inc., Chicago, IL.

● Suskind, R. M. (ed.) (1977) *Malnutrition and the Immune Response*. Raven Press, N.Y.

[6] McDougall, J. A. and M. A. McDougall (1983) *The McDougall Plan*. New Century Publishers, Inc. Piscataway, N.J. See pp. 116–122 for an extensive review of the scientific literature on the relationship between fiber-deficient diets and gastrointestinal disorders.

[7] Ornish, D. (1983) "Effects of stress management training and dietary changes in treating ischemia heart disease," *JAMA* 249: 54

[8] Bernard, J. (1981) "Effects of an intensive, short-term exercise and

nutrition program on patients with coronary heart disease," *J Card Rehab* 1: 99

[9] Gershwin, M. E. et al. (1985) *Nutrition and Immunity*: "In vivo effects of fatty acids" Academic Press, N.Y.

[10] Beisel, W. R. et al. (1981) "Single-nutrient effects on immunologic functions." *J. Am. Med. Assoc.* 245(1): 53–58

[11] Gershwin, M. E. et al. (1985) Op cit.

[12] Wurtman, R. J. and J. H. Growdon (1980) "Diet enhancement of central nervous system neurotransmitters", in: *Neuroendocrinology*. Sinauer Associates, Inc., Sunderland, MA. pp. 59–60

[13] Fernstrom, J. D. (1979) "How food affects your brain." *Nutrition Action Newsletter*. December. pp. 5–7

[14] Schwartz, G. (1979) "Foodstuffs of the brain." in: *Food Power*. McGraw-Hill Book Co. N.Y. pp. 55–58

[15] Benton, M. (1985) "Can a vegetarian diet make you mellow?" *Vegetarian Times*, June. pp. 17–18

[16] Benton, M. (1985) Ibid.

[17] Hewitt, W. (1975) "Clinical implications of the presence of drug residues in food," *Fed Proc*. 34: 202

[18] Fairweather, F. (1981) "Food additives and cancer," *Proc. Nutr. Soc.* 40: 21

[19] Howe, G. (1977) "Artificial sweetener and human bladder cancer," *Lancet* 2: 578

[20] National Academy of Sciences (1982) *Diet, Nutrition, and Cancer*. Washington D.C., N.A.S. Special report on diet and cancer. 472 pages

[21] Rosenbaum, M. (1984) Op cit. p. 98

[22] Krishnan, S. *et al*. (1974) "Effect of vitamin A and protein-calorie undernutrition on immune responses." *Immunology* 28: 383

[23] Chandra, R. K. and B. Au, (1981) "Single nutrient deficiency and cell-mediated immune responses." III vitamin A. *Nutr Res*. 1: 181

[24] Nauss, K. M. *et al*. (1979) "The effect of vitamin A deficiency on the in vitro cellular immune response of rats." *J. Nutr*. 109: 1815

[25] Chandra, R. K. and B. Au, (1981) Op. Cit.

[26] Goldfarb, R. H. and R. B. Herberman (1981) "Natural killer cell reactivity: regulatory interactions among phorbol ester, interferon, cholera toxin and retinoic acid." *J. Immunol*. 126: 2129

[27] Dennert, G. and R. Lotan (1978) "Effects of retinoic acid on the immune system: stimulation of T-killer cell induction." *Eur. J. Immunol*. 8: 23

[28] Dennert, G. *et al*. (1979) "Retinoic acid stimulation of the induction of mouse killer T-cell in allogeneic and syngeneic systems." *J. Natl Cancer Inst*. 62: 89

[29] Malkovsky, M. *et al*. (1983) "T-cell mediated enhancement of host-versus-graft reactivity in mice fed a diet enriched in vitamin A acetate." *Nature* 302: 338

[30] Cranton, E. M. and J. P. Frackelton (1984) "Free radical pathology in age-associated disease: treatment with EDTA chelation, nutrition and antioxidants." *J. Hol. Med.* 6(1): 6–38

[31] Kutsky, R. J. (1981) Op. Cit. p. 233

[32] Posner, B. M., Broitman, S. A. and Vitale, J. J. (1980) "Nutrition in neoplastic disease." from: *Advances in Modern Human Nutrition and Dietetics* 29: 130–169.

[33] Beisel, W. R. *et al.* (1981) Op cit.

[34] Axelrod, A. E. (1971) Op Cit.

[35] Beisel, W. R. *et al.* (1981) Op cit.

[36] Beisel, W. R. *et al.* (1981) Op cit.

[37] Posner, B. M. *et al.* (1980) Op cit.

[38] Axelrod, A. E. (1971) "Immune processes in vitamin deficiency states." *Am. J. Clin. Nutr.* 24: 265

[39] Kutsky, R. J. (1981) Op cit. pp. 219, 228

[40] Sakane, T. *et al.* (1982) "Effects of methyl-B12 on the *in vitro* immune functions of human T lymphocytes." *J. Clin Immunol* 2: 101

[41] Beisel, W. (1981) Op cit.

[42] Kutsky, R. J. (1981) Op cit. pp. 242–251

[43] Gershwin, M. E. *et al.* eds. (1985) Op cit. p. 254

[44] Thomas, W. R. and P. G. Holt (1978) "Vitamin C and immunity: an assessment of the evidence." *Clin. Exp. Immunol.* 32: 370–9

[45] McCarty, M. F. (1982) "Nutritional insurance supplementation and corticosteroid toxicity." *Med. Hypothesis* 9: 15–156

[46] Newberne, P. M. and V. Suphakarn (1983) "Nutrition and cancer: a review, with emphasis on the role of vitamins C and E and selenium." *Nutrition and Cancer* 5: 107–118

[47] Germann, D. R. (1977) *The Anti-Cancer Diet.* Wyden Books, Ridgefield, CT.

[48] Kutsky, R. J. (1981) Op. cit. p. 253

[49] Gershwin, M. E. *et al.* (1985) Op. cit. p. 244

[50] Beisel, W. R. *et al.* (1981) Op cit.

[51] Beisel, W. R. *et al.* (1981) Ibid.

[52] Harris, R. S. and K. Thimann, eds. (1967–1976) "Vitamins and hormones." Volumes 25–34. Academic Press, N.Y.

[53] Beach, R. S., Gershwin, M. E. and L. S. Hurley (1982) "Zinc, copper, and manganese in immune function and experimental oncogenesis." *Nutrition and Cancer* 3: 172

[54] Gershwin, M. E. *et al.* (1985) Op cit. p. 209

[55] Cunninham-Rundles *et al.* (1980) Op cit.   ** In Gershwin

[56] Beisel, (1976)   ** In Gershwin.

[57] Kutsky, R. J. (1981) Op cit. p. 125

[58] McCarty, M. F. (1982) "Nutritional insurance supplementation and corticosteroid toxicity." *Medical Hypotheses* 9: 15

[59] Gershwin, M. E. *et al.* (1985) Op cit. p. 201–204

[60] Beach, R. S., Gershwin, M. E. and L. S. Hurley (1982) Op cit.

[61] Chandra, R. K. (1981) "Immunocompetence as a function of nutritional status." *Brit Med. Bull.* 37: 89

[62] Gershwin, M. E. *et al.* (1985) Op. cit. p. 222

[63] Milanino *et al.* (1979)   ** In Gershwin

[64] Baker and Jultquist (1978)   ** In Gershwin

[65] Kollman, D. (1986) Biochemist and nutritional consultant. (Personal communications.) Cell Tech, Inc. Klamath Lake; Oregon.

[66] Ballentine, R. (1979) Op cit. pp. 23–38; 223–278

[67] Schroeder, H. (1974) *The Poisons Around Us.* University Press, Bloomington, IN, p. 126

[68] Tashev, T. (1981) "Nutrition and chronic disease. "A. E. Harper & G. K. Davis (eds.); Alan R. Liss, Inc. N.Y., N.Y.

[69] Underwood, E. (1977) *Trace Elements in Human and Animal Nutrition* 4th ed. Academic Press, N.Y. p. 267

[70] Kutsky, R. J. (1981) Op cit. pp. 216–220

[71] Gershwin *et al.* (1983)   ** Find ref in Gershwin

[72] Klevay *et al.* (1979)   ** In Gershwin

[73] Klevay *et al.* (1979) Ibid.

[74] Pfeiffer, C. (1975) *Mental and Elemental Nutrients.*   ** from AIDS book

[75] Anderson, B. (1981) "The iron and zinc status of long-term vegetarian women." *Am. J. Clin.Nutr.* 34: 1042

[76] Dossey, L. (1982) "Time symmetry and asymmetry," in: *Space, Time, and Medicine.* Shambhala Publications, Inc., London. pp. 165–6

A Macrobiotic View of Healing

Marc Van Cauwenberghe, M.D.

he word "medicine" is derived from the Latin word *medire*, hich means "to walk in the middle." A "remedy" is therefore something that brings us back to the middle." The word "doctor" riginated in *docere* or "to teach." So, a "medical doctor" was riginally "someone who studied and taught how to find the iddle." To find the middle, we must know where the extremities e. The study of extremities (yin and yang) and the middle is the aracteristic feature of macrobiotics. A macrobiotic teacher is erefore fully involved in "medicine" in its original sense.

The word "hospital" is derived from *domus hospitalis*, meaning house of a host," or "hospitable home." In this home one could nd *therapeuts*, originally meaning "servants," or "caretakers." "clinic" was nothing but a place where someone went to rest *linein:* "to recline or lie down"). A "recovery" consisted of ceiving a "new cover," meaning new blood, tissues, and perhaps udy and discussion. This is precisely the way we take care of our ealth and deal with health-related problems in macrobiotics.

Discovering Macrobiotics

fter my mother's death I got a week off. I used it for my favor-e hobby at that time: browsing in second-hand bookstores. I truck upon a privately published, stenciled, badly translated ablication titled *Cancer and the Philosophy of the Far East* by eorge Ohsawa.[1] "Interesting title," I thought . . . .

Struggling through the book I managed to understand its main lea: A human being is a creator ("God created man in His

Presently published as *The Macrobiotic Way of Healing* by the George Ohsawa Macrobiotic Foundation, Oroville, California.

image"). He cannot escape this fact. Every day he has to rebuild, re-create himself (strangely, nowadays re-creation has a quite different and in practice often an opposite meaning). This minimum necessary and actually sufficient tool for this re-creation is food: air, water, solid foods. Air we take more or less instinctively. Over water we have more control: we can decide to drink more than our thirst demands. But solid foods generate a vast number of decisions for us: what substances are most suitable to daily re-create and fuel a human being's organs and functions? How much food to take? In what proportions? How to prepare it?

To help us make these most important decisions, we do not need a continuously changing dietary science, Ohsawa said. What we need is a knowledge of the order of the universe, or the principle of yin and yang. Animals instinctively know this principle. Humans know it when they are embryos, and through it build their wonderful body. Young children know it and owe their keen curiosity to it. But we start to suppress our awareness of this universal principle as we fill ourselves with concepts, artificial education, hypotheses, and all types of knowledge which have nothing to do with life. All of us, though, retain our awareness of yin and yang some degree: we can distinguish hot from cold, left from right. If not, then our life is constantly in danger. Because we clouded our awareness of yin and yang, most of us cannot clearly, simply, and immediately answer the request to define concepts such as love, truth, peace, happiness, and freedom. Thus we have hundreds of contradictory philosophies and religions.

Ohsawa stated that man must recover his intuitive understanding of the Order of Creation, his "unclouded judging ability." How to do this? Read Lao Tze, or the *I Ching*? If we do this with our present conceptual mind, we will misinterpret these works, miss their main points, and may start to devote our life to conceptual accentuation of selected aspects of them, or splinter them into hundreds of conflicting religious and spiritual movements. George Ohsawa warns not to read these or any other works over and over understand the principle of yin and yang, or the order of the universe. And after acquiring this understanding. we do not need to read them anymore; we could write an updated version using today's vocabulary and preoccupations to illustrate our point.

How, then, to recover our intuition. Ohsawa said that this could be accomplished simply by eating according to the order of the universe, or nature. Such a way of eating was not invented by Ohsawa. It was practiced and described in ancient cultures and religions around the world. When societies abandoned this dietary practice (usually after becoming wealthy), they started to decline and eventually vanished, or stayed alive as a living corpse.

But this concept must be approached with common sense. The way of eating prescribed in the Bible, for example, was suitable for populations in the biblical countries, and during biblical times. To eat in exactly the same way now, in any country, would be nonsense. Besides, the Eskimo, and other peoples living in extreme climates, could not follow such recommendations at all.

We must see the "why" of these dietary prescriptions. The reasoning behind them is based on an application of the principle of yin and yang. These opposite and complementary tendencies can be interpreted as the "two hands of God" through which everything comes into existence. If we understand why and how these hands originate, what they represent, and how they interact with each other, we understand life, creation, the whole universe.

I later discovered that *Cancer and the Philosophy of the Far East* was Ohsawa's last major book; it was his conclusion, after having written some 150 books, and enough letters and magazine articles to fill another 150 volumes.

Although the book still gave me the feeling of a fairy tale, I found enough in it to give his hypothesis a chance and started to experiment with it. I was fortunate to love immediately all the foods he had recommended. Without really expecting it, three weeks later my skin ailments were GONE, and my intestines were at peace.

Soon I also started to discover people who had known Ohsawa and had recovered from such problems as stomach cancer, chronic bronchitis, allergies, rheumatoid arthritis, epilepsy, leukemia, and other illnesses through his recommendations.

Having now practiced, taught, and recommended macrobiotics for eighteen years, I agree with Ohsawa that opposition to the order of nature is ultimately rooted in our greediness, distrustfulness, discrimination, and lack of curiosity, wonder, and appreciation: in one word, in the ultimate disease from which all so-called diseases are but a symptom: egotism. He saw cancer as a full-blown manifestation of all kinds of egotistical thoughts and the behaviors derived from them.

One of the oldest books in the world is *The Yellow Emperor's Classic of Internal Medicine* (1000 B.C.). In the first chapter, the Yellow Emperor asks a doctor: "In ancient times people lived over a hundred years, yet remained active. Nowadays people reach only half that age and become decrepit. Why is that?" The doctor answered, "People understood the order of the universe (Tao) and patterned themselves upon the yin and the yang. There was temperance in eating and drinking."

In Mayan medicine a physician would not prescribe any specific remedies, such as herbs, without advising the patient to eat only corn for ten days. After all, didn't God create man out of corn?

Hippocrates is considered to be the founder of the art of medicine. In my opinion, he was standing at its ending. After him medicine became less and less of an art; it became fragmented, and forgot its main issue. Before Hippocrates, medicine didn't need to be written down and categorized: medicine was built into people's lifestyle itself. That lifestyle was macrobiotics. The Order of Creation was called Logos. Sickness was taught to be the result of offending the "gods," which represented the various forces in nature. Ancient people deeply understood in their origin, mechanism, function, value and purpose of these forces.

Jesus wanted to remind people about macrobiotics. He stated that all diseases can be handled by "prayer" and "fasting." That is to say: macrobiotics. But don't be misled. Fasting and prayer do not mean abstaining from food while uttering the Lord's Prayer repeatedly with a solemn voice. "Fasting" means to take only the necessary amounts of absolutely necessary food. In Jesus' time that was whole grain bread and water. This regimen is particularly effective when one has generally been eating "orderly," but indulged and thereby created sickness. For people eating far outside macrobiotic guidelines, consuming only with exotic foods, refined foods, animal foods, and the like, a fast should include grains, beans, land and sea vegetables, local fruits, and maybe small amounts of fish: the standard macrobiotic diet.

"Prayer" is nothing but reawakening the spirit of self-reflection, the attitude of responsibility, an appreciation for natural foods, a sense of apology toward the body one has abused, outstretched, overstimulated, intoxicated, or neglected. One can thereby happily and thankfully practice a macrobiotic way of eating. We could say that prayer is seeing the whole picture.

According to our inclination we can start with one or the other or both of these factors. Interestingly, as we "fast," "prayers" arise more and more spontaneously; and as we "pray" this way, fasting will follow naturally. If people have trouble "sticking to the diet" (which is a misconception about macrobiotic practice), it is because this "praying" attitude has not been reawakened yet.

This kind of fasting and praying is sufficient to handle problems when we are living macrobiotically. For others, additional help can be found in shiatsu, compresses and plasters, or some specific food preparation.

Ohsawa formulated his views about living in harmony with nature in the late 1920s, and used the Japanese expression *Sei-Shoku* ("correct nourishment") to describe them. In a book written in French in 1952, the *Book of Judo*, he stated: "My method is a kind of macrobiotics," borrowing the word from the German physician, Hufeland, who used it to describe a method for securing a long and healthy life. Later, while reading in Europe and the United States, Ohsawa started to use the word "macrobiotics" to describe the way to develop a healthy, free, and happy life.

In 1959 Ohsawa wrote his first book in English. He wanted to call it *Macrobiotics: The Biology and Physiology of Zen*. At that time Zen philosophy was becoming popular, and Ohsawa wanted to state that trying to understand and practice Zen without establishing the biological and physiological foundation upon which Zen grew can only lead to partial understanding. For a reason unknown to me, he changed the title to *Zen Macrobiotics*, a strange expression, although his French translation of this book is called *Le Zen Macrobiotique* (Macrobiotic Zen). He was definitely more fluent in French than in English.

Anybody who thinks critically would probably agree that recovery cannot be achieved by surgically removing or by paralyzing a sickness. At that time a sickness has been destroyed, not a patient healed. Even if we kill bacteria, the patient has not yet recovered. Why couldn't he cope with the bacteria? Medical doctors may say, "Because he didn't have the necessary antibodies." Macrobiotics would say, "Because he was an excellent food source for those bacteria." Don't bacteria grow well on jams, fruits, milk products, meats, potatoes, and moist foods?

Traditional ways of preserving meats were drying and pickling. To "preserve" our cells and tissues, it is better to not take more liquid than our body requires through thirst, and to use salt wisely —both too much and too little will cause imbalance. Salt is so powerful that it creates problems when taken excessively, particularly in combination with excess liquid, meat, eggs, cheese, and so on. But if used macrobiotically, salt supplies us with the best immunity against micro-organisms. In 1956, in Lambarene, Gabon, Ohsawa recovered, in thirty days, from tropical ulcers, which were then 100 percent lethal. To do this he used macrobiotic preparations cooked with the necessary amounts of salt.

In my opinion, only a person, and not a sickness, can be healed. To be healed means that one can take care of his health. It does not mean that he never becomes sick. We become sick because we do not maintain balance in our bodies, and between our bodies and the environment. Both are continuously changing and balance must be dynamically re-established every day. This sounds more difficult than it is. We do the same sort of balancing, on a moment-by-moment basis, when we ride a bike.

To be healthy through macrobiotics can therefore not be achieved by rigidly applying a set of food rules. It can only be realized through an artful, playful application of the universal principles of life in one's day-to-day living. This is also how animals in the wild keep enjoying the best health and cure themselves if and when they become sick.

In this light it is totally out of the question to declare either a disease or a patient as incurable. The doctor can only declare:

"I am sorry, I am unable to treat this disease," or "I cannot cure you. . . ."

Many people drawn to macrobiotics are already in a more or less deep state of sickness, and their dietary patterns are far from macrobiotic recommendations. It is therefore not surprising to see big changes in their physical and psychological condition after they start to shift their diet. They may change their mind as often as they have to change the size of their pants. This however is transitory. While their previous body fades, a new body of different quality is arising; it may take several years to appear: this largely depends on their skill in preparing the foods, their chewing efforts, their digestive capacity, and steadiness in practicing.

I would like to summarize my observations in regard to healing through macrobiotics:

1. There are no sicknesses, but only sick people. I started to realize this in medical school, but then went right along studying diseases only and seeing people as "cases."

2. Unless a person wants to change towards macrobiotics, "putting someone on a macrobiotic diet" can be only temporarily successful. He usually abandons his "diet" sooner or later.

3. In patients taking responsibility and making the necessary efforts, I have seen all types of diseases vanish, including "incurable ones," using solely macrobiotic food preparations and way of life suggestions. Some examples include: Crohn's disease, endometriosis, rheumatoid arthritis, migraines, lupus erythematosus, chronic bladder infections, chronic bronchitis, infertility of various natures, pinched nerve, and others.

4. If despite the person's efforts the disease did not vanish, the following were often the reasons:

    a) He had already been heavily altered in some way (multiple operations, drug treatments for many years).

    b) His surroundings (family, friends, physician) were antagonizing or sabotaging him.

    c) He was involved in difficult personal situations (divorce, financial pressure, unhappy relationships) and wasn't actually aware that they could work antagonistically.

    d) Unknowingly, he was making one or another gross

mistake. For example: a woman improved very quickly from multiple sclerosis, then started worsening; this relapse coincided with her starting to use an electric blanket, and she didn't suspect this at all to be the cause.

Ten years ago I witnessed an osteosarcoma vanish from the knee of a young woman. I wondered how I could prove the validity of macrobiotics through this case. Consulting a professor of epidemiology, I was told: "Find a similar case—the same age and sex—and achieve the same result through the same advice." I didn't even start to look for such a "case." I do not usually give the same advice, even to two people with apparently similar conditions. Everyone is different and therefore needs different advice. Even if I had found such a person, and the advice turned out to be similar, her understanding, situation, intensity of wanting to heal, and ability to enjoy macrobiotics would be different, and the result might therefore not be the same.

A macrobiotic person does not oppose, antagonize, or reject the modern medical approach. But he also does not want to be forced, threatened, or scared into using it. If a modern medical treatment becomes necessary, he wants to take advantage of this method only after discussion with the doctor he selected, and after looking into all possible alternatives.

A macrobiotic person therefore takes responsibility for having created his disease, having chosen his physician, and having accepted his line of treatment.

If I would choose to work as a regular physician for the macrobiotic people in the world, I might starve, because of a lack of clients. My purpose as a macrobiotic teacher is simple: to make my job obsolete. After that I would like to be a singing poet or stand-up comedian, although I doubt whether the world would have a need for this—everybody might want to have such a profession. So most probably I would become a farmer, baker, house builder, plumber, weaver, or something similar.

I Enjoy Macrobiotics

I enjoy natural foods more than any other. They are superior in quality, taste, and artistic composition. Most other foods and food preparations feel like a lie to me. Most breads only look like bread, ice cream is but an extremely ephemeral ghost, and white sugar is a lie because it doesn't really exist as such in nature. If we are what we eat, what do we really create by consuming those products? Can we call "food" items which create sickness, cancer, rigid thinking, anger, fear, misery?

When I smell or see dairy foods, I can sense the sadness of the cow and calf in them. Eggs and chicken remind me of concentration camps. Steaks of blood, slaughter, horror, fear.

I admire the humbleness of grains, beans, sea and land vegetables, and sea salt, waiting to be consumed as they are. They are beautiful in their simplicity. They do not need to be polished.

All you have to do discover whether a "food" is really a food, is chew it very well. Chew a mouthful of rice one hundred times and then try the same with chicken, cheese, meat. Chew whole grain sourdough bread and compare it with chewing croissants or white bread. You may taste the difference between health and sickness, truth and lie, joy and sadness, happiness and unhappiness, life and death.

Most people think that using medications or inventing new technologies is the shortest way towards health. Generally people prefer shortcuts. Taking this route many find out that it actually didn't bring them where they wanted to go. Their general health worsens, the task of re-creating it seems to become bigger and bigger, and the chances of achieving well-being seem to become dimmer and dimmer.

The way to establish freedom from disease cannot include shortcuts, such as taking vaccinations. Vaccinations may already set us out on the road toward degenerative and infectious diseases that we have no vaccinations for. People who think that their lives are more protected if they wear a gun are making the same mistake. Their fearful attitude and distrust itself emanates an odor that is very attractive to possible muggers; and their constant fear wears down their nervous system and endocrine glands.

Macrobiotics may seem like the long way, because it involves self-training and development of one's understanding, but there is no shortcut to health. We cannot grow from baby to adulthood in a couple of days. Taking recreational drugs will not accelerate the development of spirituality. However, of all natural and necessarily long ways to health and spirituality, macrobiotics offers the shortest way. Each day of practicing macrobiotics offers results, whether we notice them or not.

Macrobiotics is actually an endless way. There is no end in improving our health, understanding, and freedom. We might even say that macrobiotics is no way, and therefore the only true way. Eating grains is not a way to health: without using grains humanity would never have evolved, and therefore humanity has no other way to sustain itself.

If we don't judge from the perspective of the order of the universe, then what is short seems long to us, what is long seems short. All "short" ways (surgery, injections, etc.) were the result of enormously long, expensive experimentations on countless animals and people by numerous researchers. Instant foods were not invented in a day. All "long" ways are actually short. They were discovered in the daily lives of our ancestors. The practice of eating grains and beans didn't have to be invented at all by humans are the result of it. Eating such foods is therefore really the shortest way or no way; it is only common sense, just as it is common sense to breathe.

A Self-Critique by a Doctor Trained in Modern Medicine

Looking back on how I used to think about and deal with health and sickness, I realize the following:

1. Basically I had acquired an aggressive attitude. Based on the presumption that in life "a struggle for survival" is going on, and judging that my life or human life is of high value, I had no doubts about using an arsenal of weapons to deal with

everything I saw as invader or aggressor, although these were also manifestations of life.

Through macrobiotics I learned that our "enemy" is our benefactor, and that he can be turned into our best friend. Since practicing macrobiotics not even a mosquito has been bothering me.

I now realize that this paranoid, aggressive, militaristic attitude was fed by the consumption of animal products (particularly meat and eggs).

I thought that life is a complex biochemical phenomenon that can run berserk. The more details I became informed of, the more this view was supported. There was no chance for exploring other possibilities. I had enough to do with assimilating the complexities of this particular approach.

This acceptance of seeing things in a fragmented, purely analytical, complicated way came about and was enhanced by eating refined foods (white flour products and sugar), heavily processed foods, chemicalized' foods, fragmented foods (for example, only part of a fruit), and a total lack of simple, wholesome, central food in my diet.

I thought that I was thinking. When Michio Kushi asked me to simply but comprehensively define love, peace, freedom, happiness, truth, health, sickness, life. I could only quote from books, and I didn't wonder why I couldn't find good definitions in encyclopedias or why I myself couldn't come up with an acceptable response. I thought that answering these questions was the unique capacity and right of philosophical giants.

The amount and depth of my philosophical study during medical school was extremely limited: only some Western philosophers were summarized and Aristotelian-based logic was explained. I now fully realize the shallowness of thinking that such schooling produces. We can only define in incomplete, vague, or complicated ways, and often the outcomes vary from day to day. I once went to my ex-professor of philosophy and asked him for his "definition of a definition." He smiled but didn't answer. Through macrobiotics I realize that this lack of depth, ability, and precision in thinking has a lot to do with not chewing whole foods, in other words, not using our "wisdom" teeth for what they are made for: thoroughly grinding whole grains. By eating whole foods and chewing well, we notice that we start to seek and see a whole view, in which all details we carry along can beautifully be fit in. We see that Aristotelian logic is a complete mirror image of logics in terms of yin and yang, which is the dynamics of life itself, of all changes.

4. I realize that I and my colleagues carried the pride of working with the advances of modern medicine, and the naiveté that our medicine would one day control all diseases.

   Now I realize that proud people are on the verge of downfall, and that all progress not in harmony with life itself is actually a regression, or at least that every advance is accompanied by a regression. Pride and naiveté are charming juvenile attitudes, particularly enhanced by the consumption of milk, milk products, and simple sugars.

5. I was carrying the attitude that only the "scientific method" is a sensible way to investigate nature. I scorned dogmatic religious and metaphysical ways, therapy actually manifesting the same dogmatism in my field.

   What is the biological background of such dogmatism? My answer to this I leave for you to discover.

If we subconsciously or consciously carry such attitudes of aggressivity, unclarity, delusion, pride, naiveté, and fanaticism, it is only natural that we don't exercise any self-critique. We keep seeing only what we achieved (increase of life span, wiping out of this and that), but we do not always see at what price and what simultaneously resulted: increasing morbidity, arrival of more and more serious diseases, increase of life span mostly because we keep people alive longer rather than improving their health and happiness.

Since we don't criticize ourselves, critique had to come from outside. First it came from the East. This was George Ohsawa's life work. But his admonitions were not expressed in an exact language, not experimentally verifiable, not illustrated by statistics.

Until now they have had very little impact on the direction of modern medicine. Since we didn't have trust in anyone but ourselves and in our methods, how could we grant him our thoughtful consideration?

Of course, as long as one doesn't eat according to macrobiotic principles, it is difficult to comprehend or even imagine the logic and power of macrobiotics. By the same token, as long as one doesn't think more holistically, it is difficult to eat properly. Is there no way out then? According to yin and yang one can start by trying to do the opposite of what he has been doing: try to listen instead of talk, try to look at the whole instead of the part, and think "I don't know much" instead of "I know a lot." In this way, one can come to see and experience a more complete view of life.

Hope for the Future

From practicing and teaching macrobiotics for more than eighteen years, I can see how the natural way of healing can influence the future development of medicine in a positive direction. The following points emerge from this consideration:

1. *Cooperation with Nature:* Cooperation with nature has been the essence of medical practice from the beginning. Hippocrates taught that the best healer was one who interfered least with the body's natural healing ability. The body has numerous mechanisms that, when properly nourished through diet and way of living, can restore health or equilibrium. The art of healing consists of allowing these natural healing abilities to come forth by providing the proper food, home care, environment, and view of life.

Actually, it is far easier to be healthy than it is to become ill. Sickness is usually the result of many unnecessary efforts. For example, making brown rice or other whole grains available requires less time and effort than refining or polishing them. Extra capital, machinery, labor, and time are needed to convert brown rice into white rice, or whole wheat flour into refined flour. Moreover, brown rice and other whole grains contain a natural balance of minerals, protein, carbohydrate, and vitamins. They are complete, naturally balanced foods. However, white rice or other polished grains lack many of the original, essential nutrients found in their unrefined counterparts, including B-vitamins. Eating them can result in nutritional deficiencies, including beri-beri, or vitamin-B deficiency. The net result of these additional efforts is to create foods that can make us sick. It is far simpler and easier to leave the grains as they are and thereby avoid the sicknesses caused by eating refined foods.

In order to compensate for the lack of nutrients in refined foods, time, effort, and labor are used to create artificial vitamins. An entire industry has developed because we are interfering with the natural nutritional balance in our foods. If we left them as they were, all of this time and energy could be diverted into other, more useful pursuits.

Feeding babies artificial formulas offers another example. The ideal, naturally balanced food for newborns is mother's milk. It is available at no cost and requires no additional efforts to produce. However, instead of simply using this wonderful natural food, we try to feed babies with the milk of cows. This requires tremendous additional and unnecessary efforts. Because cow's milk is not suited to humans, but to baby cows, we must tamper with it in order to make it nutritionally tolerable. Still, even with the addition of sugar or other substances, it can never be as ideal as mother's milk. Moreover, a variety of unpleasant side effects are produced in the babies who are fed this artificially engineered substance. Digestive upsets, allergies, frequent colds, flu, and infections, and many other chronic and acute problems result from cow's-milk formulas, problems that are far less common or nonexistent among breast-fed babies. Then, more efforts are required to deal with these side effects, some of which, such as antibiotics and other medications, create additional side effects in an endless cycle of cause and effect. Even though these practices are common in the modern world, they sound as if they were taken from Erasmus' *Praise of Folly*.

The more artificial interference we create, the more side (or counterbalancing) effects result, while the more we allow nature to work by itself, the fewer side effects are produced. These side

ffects may be immediately apparent, as they are in the case of
arious types of chemotherapy and other medications, or may be
ubtle and long term. For example, although removing the tonsils
ay relieve the immediate symptoms of tonsilitis, in the long run
 weakens the body's natural immune ability and capacity to
ischarge toxic excess. Often, when some future problem develops,
e miss the connection between it and a past procedure such as
moving the tonsils. We must become wise observers and re-
ember that everything is interconnected and every unnatural
rocedure will cause some type of side effect, either immediately
r in the future.

The understanding of yin and yang, or the way that comple-
entary/antagonistic factors work in nature and in the human
ody can help us to see this interconnectedness more clearly. In
e traditional medicine of the Far East, for example, which is
ased on this principle, the major organs in the body are classified
to complementary pairs. This classification, which dates back
t least as far as the *Yellow Emperor's Classic*, is as follows:

More Yang (Compact, Solid) Organs	*More Yin (Hollow, Expanded) Organs*
Liver	Gallbladder
Heart	Small Intestine
Spleen (Pancreas)	Stomach
Lungs	Large Intestine
Kidney	Bladder

Problems of dysfunction in any of the organs are accompanied
y related dysfunction in the complementary partner. As we can
e, if we operate on or remove an organ or part of an organ, we
lso effect its complementary partner, as well as the body as a
hole, including the person's mental and emotional condition.
Not only are the organs and other parts of the body functioning
gether as an integrated whole, but so are the mind, body, and
motions.

In my experience, it is far wiser to first try the most natural
ethods—such as balanced diet and simple home care—that carry

practically no risk of side effects, before proceeding to more drasti
or invasive procedures that can cause a multitude of side effects

2.   Encouraging Independence and Responsibility: Health is th
responsibility of each person. Therefore, in the future, it is my hop
that medicine will guide everyone in the direction of greater re
sponsibility for their own health, rather than encouraging depend
ence on others. Our day-to-day actions—including our diet, type o
exercise, activity, and other behaviors—are the primary factor
that determine health or sickness. No one, not our doctor
lawyer, psychiatrist, minister, or rabbi, can take this responsibilit'
for us. No one can chew or exercise for us. Taking responsibilit'
for our health and our life is the first step toward maturity and
genuine freedom.

3.   Education is the Best Medicine: In the future, I hope tha
medicine will shift from an emphasis on the treatment of disease
after they develop to preventing them from developing in the firs
place. Education is therefore necessary to equip people with the
knowledge and practical skills they need to maintain their health
Medicine must begin to address basic questions such as what is
the proper way of living as a human being on this planet, including
the most ideal way of eating, and concern itself with practica
issues such as chewing, cooking, and orienting daily life in a positive direction. Practical advice and guidance, grounded in aware
ness of natural order, are what is needed, rather than conceptua
theories. The way to be healthy should be practical and simple
and easily understood by everyone. It should ideally become par
of everyone's intuitive common sense, and not require specialized
knowledge. It therefore cannot be the exclusive province or
monopoly of any one group or elite class, but part of the common
knowledge and daily life of everyone.

4.   Conserving Our Resources: Actually, a healthful life is the
most economical and least wasteful. For example, many observers
have noted how expensive modern medical treatments have be
come, and how a shift to a naturally balanced preventive die
could result in substantial savings (please see *Choice for Survival*
The Baby Boomer's Dilemma by Edward Kelly and Ralph Kidder

apan Publications, 1988). In *Dietary Goals for the United States*, ssued by the U.S. Senate Select Committee on Nutrition and Iuman Needs, for example, the potential for cost savings resultig from dietary improvements were discussed as follows:

> In testimony before the Select Committee in 1972, Dr. George Briggs, professor of nutrition at the University of California, Berkeley, estimated, based on a study by the Department of Agriculture, that improved nutrition might cut the nation's health bill by one-third. The Department of Health, Education and Welfare's *Forward Plan for Health*, *FY 1978–82*, reports that health care expenditures in the United States in Fiscal Year 1975 totalled about $118.5 billion and predicts the cost could exceed $230 billion by Fiscal Year 1980.

Today, medical costs are much higher than this, and if we factor 1 potential costs of treating a problem such as AIDS, the cost of 1edical treatment in the future could become astronomical. In 1is case, society may have no other choice but to implement low-ost, natural healthcare strategies, especially the macrobiotic diet 1d way of life.

The cost of high-tech medicine is especially increasing, including rocedures such as organ- and bone-marrow transplants. It is far ss expensive to strengthen the natural function of the organs 1rough natural diet, and prevent their deterioration, than do 1thing until the degenerative process reaches the point where the ·gans can no longer function and have to be replaced.

The Medicine of Humanity

1 the future, it is my hope that medicine will emphasize health .ther than sickness. For this a practical definition of health—such that developed by George Ohsawa and Michio Kushi—will rve us well. These points illustrate how health is a far more /namic process than just the avoidance of disease: health is :tually the joyful process of living on this earth. The conditions ˙ health as taught in macrobiotics include:*

From the *Book of Macrobiotics: the Universal Way of Health, Happiness and Peace* by Michio Kushi with Alex Jack, Japan Publications, 1986.

1. Never Be Tired
2. Have a Good Appetite
3. Have Good Sleep
4. Have Good Memory
5. Never Be Angry
6. Be Joyous and Alert
7. Have Endless Appreciation

In traditional Oriental medicine, which is many thousands of years old, three levels of doctors were identified. The first, or lowest grade doctor, dealt only with the symptoms of disease, adjusting imbalance in the body with technique such as herbal medicine, acupuncture, therapeutic massage, or others. In any case, he or she dealt only with the presenting symptoms themselves.

Middle grade doctors were more concerned with the underlying causes of sickness. Although they understood how to use the symptomatic approaches mentioned above, they saw behind symptoms and realized that other factors were actually causing the patient to become ill. Inevitably, he or she understood that the patient's diet, lifestyle, and view of life were in dis-order. Advice was therefore more educational and directed toward helping the patient self-reflect and change the underlying causes of the sickness.

The highest grade doctor went beyond individual sicknesses and into the realm of social problems. He or she guided individuals and humanity as a whole toward health and well-being by teaching how to return to the middle way and live in harmony with nature. In this sense, he or she was more of a philosopher or educator than a physician. Ultimately, this type of doctor could resolve various conflicts between individuals and groups within society. He or she had the ability to establish peace and harmony between the parts of the body, for the benefit of the body as a whole, and between parts of society, for the benefit of humanity as a whole. In the future, the medicine of humanity will share a similar goal by reaching beyond the treatment of individual sicknesses and toward the establishment of a healthy and peaceful world.

My Explorations in Macrobiotics

Henry Edward Altenberg, M.D.

I have been a physician for forty years, specializing in child and family psychiatry. At the age of sixty-two, however, I am a newcomer to macrobiotics. I began following a predominantly macrobiotic diet one year ago. At this point I can only offer preliminary thoughts and observations. I consider myself a freshman student and participant. The reason for my initial interest grew out of being given a diagnosis of thyroid tumor in May of 1986.

I had consulted my family physician because of a distinctly unpleasant stiff neck on the right side, which had persisted for about two weeks. I had had rare twinges of discomfort before, and one similar episode of a stiff neck thirty-three years earlier, when I was in the Air Force during the Korean War, and stationed in Alaska as a psychiatrist. X-rays at that time showed some early evidence of osteo-arthritis.

The family doctor advised me to take some mild pain-killer and apply some heat to my right neck. He also suggested some x-rays of the cervical spine. He then performed a routine procedure, unrelated to the cervical arthritis. He placed his hands around my throat from behind and asked me to swallow, in order to check the thyroid gland. He reported that he could feel a very slight enlargement on the left side. He ordered a thyroid x-ray scan, in which a small pill of radioactive substance is swallowed, and x-rays are taken six hours and twenty-four hours later. An ultrasound examination of the thyroid was also performed with the scan. Both the scan and the ultrasound examination showed an egg-sized tumor in the left thyroid lobe. I was then referred to a surgeon for further action.

During the same week in which I had the x-rays and also saw the surgeon, I went to a local health food store, not quite knowing what I wanted. There I found a copy of *Recalled By Life* by Anthony J. Sattilaro, M.D. I also spoke with another customer who had been eating macrobiotically for about ten years. She recommended Aveline Kushi's newest cookbook, *Complete Guide to Macrobiotic Cooking*. My knowledge about macrobiotics prior to this point was miniscule. I had been aware of Erewhon products, and remembered eating at the Seventh Inn in Boston in 1976, when someone pointed out that a gentleman at one of the tables was Michio Kushi, but I did not know much about him.

The surgeon performed a needle biopsy in his office two days after the x-ray diagnosis. The following week the surgeon reported that.he could not tell if the tumor was friendly or mischievous. I was then scheduled for surgery in two weeks. The arthritis, in the meantime, began to simmer down, as predicted by the family physician, who said an acute episode often tends to be self-limiting. The x-rays of the spine did show advanced arthritis, with a "military spine," a straightening of the neck with a loss of the normal curvature which should resemble a question mark.

The surgery consisted of removal of the left lobe and isthmus of the thyroid, with the right lobe remaining. This went quite smoothly and I was out of the hospital in three days. I began to cook some of the basic recipes gleaned from the cookbook. I have enjoyed Japanese and other Oriental foods for many years, usually in restaurants. I had also started to do some modest gourmet cooking in recent years. My previous repertoire had consisted mainly of scrambled eggs and hamburgers. I found the challenge of macrobiotic cooking an enjoyable adventure. I also had become less and less of a meat consumer over the past ten or fifteen years, and had started to be more conscious of cholesterol-containing foods and fats in the past three years.

I received details from the surgeon a few weeks after surgery about the thyroid tumor. It was a relatively rare type, and a rather paradoxical one. It was not a cancer, or *carcinoma*, and yet it was not a totally friendly *adenoma*. Adenomas are usually harmless unless the space they occupy causes abnormal pressure or damage to surrounding tissues. Some of the microscopic appearance of my tumor was reported as showing a minimal degree of invasiveness, but yet not to the degree that it could qualify as a true carcinoma; therefore it was called an *invasive adenoma*.

The invasiveness was confined and limited, so there was no evidence of any true invasion! Truly a paradox: like some mythological animal with the head of one animal and the body of another, a gryphon or sphinx. This seemed to say I was, and was not, a cancer patient. Nonetheless it appeared to be a clear warning from Universal Intelligence, or God, to become healthier, and to do what I could to maintain health. The arthritis had been a strange gift which led me to obtain a very early diagnosis of the tumor, and at the same time was more than a warning, but a manifest condition. Thus I had at least two reasons for pursuing macrobiotics, cervical arthritis and the recent presence of a thyroid tumor. A third reason grew out of my interest in preventing heart disease. My father died at fifty-one, over forty years ago, of hypertensive heart disease. My oldest brother developed coronary heart disease at fifty-six and recently underwent coronary bypass surgery at sixty-six. My one other older brother has been found to have asymptomatic coronary disease.

My blood cholesterol levels have never been considered abnormal by any physician over the past twenty-five years, but I have been increasingly concerned in recent years because they were high in my opinion, and this is now supported by the reports coming out of the Framingham Study, which clearly shows significant increase in risk for heart disease if the blood cholesterol is over 200, and especially if over 250, even for persons over forty years of age. And so, I launched myself into a macrobiotic diet.

In July of 1986 my wife and I attended the *Macrobiotic Way of Life Seminar* at the Kushi Institute. About forty enrollees were present, including some spouses or companions. This was most useful, both at the theoretical and practical level. We were given lectures, cooking lessons, macrobiotic meals, and a discussion of the way of life, which is much broader than nutrition alone. We also could see what was available in books, audio and video tapes.

I also had an individual meeting with a senior dietary counselor, who interviewed me, and then suggested modifications of the standard macrobiotic diet. This included deletions or emphasis relating to the osteo-arthritis, cholesterol level, and the fact of having developed a thyroid tumor.

I began to acquire my bags of sea vegetables, numerous mason jars labeled and filled with various grains and beans, and condiments. At first I went through the classic beginner's mistakes of cooking the same dish too often, and getting somewhat discouraged or bored, as well as fantasizing about eating a banana, a tomato, or Southern fried chicken.

My initial surprise was my decreased appetite, not because I did not like the tastes, but simply because I felt full after eating grains, vegetables, and beans, without dairy or eggs and cheese. I was delighted also to lose eight or nine pounds in about six weeks and I continue to remain close to the new level. I have never been obviously overweight, and no physician has ever encouraged me to try to decrease my weight, although I have been aware that leanness is clearly healthier as one gets older. For thirty-five years I have weighed about the same 158 pounds, and am a little over five-foot seven. Like may people I have occasionally "gone on a diet" to lose weight and then discovered the commonly quoted truth that 98 percent of people regain whatever they lost within six to twelve months. In 1971 I went on the Stillman Diet and lost twelve pounds, which all returned in six months. The thought of eating such a high-protein diet today would cause me to lose my appetite easily.

Although it is still only a year since starting on a macrobiotic approach to food consumption, I remain quite optimistic about maintaining my lowered weight. Not only do I have a clearer motivation to do so, but am aware I have the tools to do so without "dieting." As I am able to be more consistent with macrobiotic principles and practices, I expect that I shall probably decrease my weight more. Overcoming a lifetime of habits and tastes, and modifying my lifestyle will probably require several years at least. Motivation and will are also important ingredients for maintaining good health. I have felt as comfortable and energetic as usual since being on the diet. I had one brief "crick" in my right neck five months ago which lasted about two days, and was very mild.

I have been studying several books about macrobiotics. There is a sizable number of volumes available from the Kushi Institute and the Ohsawa Foundation, as well as other books on nutrition that I find provocative. I see myself not only as an individual citizen with personal reasons for developing a macrobiotic approach to eating and lifestyle, but am also a professional and a student. I am curious to discover how I can competently apply it in my professional work in psychiatry and psychosomatic medicine, and perhaps bring some creative influence to bear within the medical profession. The latter hope may be somewhat grandiose at the moment, judging by some trends. Our mainstream American culture at times appears quite antithetical to healthiness and wholeness, notwithstanding jogging and aerobics. I remain an incurable optimist nonetheless. No one can easily predict changes in the rate of change.

I have not reviewed the specific content of the present-day curriculum of most medical schools of the 1980s. I suspect, however, that the demand to learn so much technological data leaves no more room for the study of prevention, health maintenance, and nutrition than was true in the 1940s when I attended medical school. A brief course in preventive medicine was required as a freshman, and this consisted mostly of reviewing public health statistics, engineering accomplishments, and socioeconomic issues. There may have been a chapter in the textbook relating to nutrition. There was no separate course in nutrition.

In obstetrics and pediatrics we did, of course, pay some attention to the role of nutrition during pregnancy. What we learned gave support to the Chinese concept of counting a person's age from the time of conception. The nine months of development is not a passive or inert process, but a vigorous interrelationship between mother and future child. When a pregnancy is relatively uneventful, little thought is given to the baby's experience as an embryo and fetus. The pregnant mother undergoes physical examinations throughout her pregnancy, and some nutritional advice is given. She is usually prescribed supplemental iron and calcium, and possibly some vitamin supplements. This is one expression of the established truth in medicine that a mother's health, illnesses, and nutrition affect her growing fetus.

The pathological impact of some drugs, medications, and toxins, especially in the first three months of pregnancy, is clearly appreciated and monitored. A significant number of useful medications can be harmful to a young fetus. In this respect nutrition is a central concern to a physician and his pregnant patient. Yet, it is also a truism that most of the time and energy of physicians are expended in more specialized attention to the diagnosis and treatment of pathological states, and only minimally to health maintenance and prevention, now as well as in the past.

In my clinical training in the third and fourth years of medical school, attention was paid to the specific dietary needs in the treatment of certain diseases, such as diabetes, liver diseases, and alcoholism, but usually as a supportive measure.

After internship and a year as a medical resident, I began my psychiatric training. The tools of the physician such as the stethoscope and ophthalmoscope were scarcely utilized, and few if any physical examinations were performed. Nutrition was even less in the consciousness of psychiatry as a field or in my training than in general medicine. Ironically, one of the most epidemic mental disorders of the early twentieth century was found to be caused by a lack of a food element, niacin, or Vitamin B_3. In the 1920s, pellagra was discovered to be due to a vitamin deficiency which caused psychosis and dementia.

Quite separate from my medical and psychiatric training and practice has been an interest for several decades in cultural anthropology and Eastern philosophy. In 1960 I began reading about Zen Buddhism, Taoism, Tibetan Buddhism, and Sufism. This also led to some partial awareness of Chinese and Oriental medicine. It came as less of a cultural shock, therefore, than it might be for some other American physicians, to learn that the *The Yellow Emperor's Classic of Internal Medicine*, the *Nei Ching*, written 5,000 years ago, might have some valid points to make about sickness and health. The ethnocentricity or cultural chauvinism of a 1980s-trained American physician can be as great as a Kalahari bushman who performs his healing ceremonies by dancing in a trance around a roaring fire, unaware of any other method to heal illness.

I speak of these interests as unplanned and unanticipated preparation for other dimensions and directions in understanding health and illness. In 1972 I read the papers presented to the first annual meeting of the American Academy of Medicine and Parapsychology. Several speakers described energy systems which were not yet defined as clearly proven within mainstream science, physics, or medicine. This included the Chinese concepts of meridians and acupuncture, the aura, and Kirlian photography. By 1974 and 1975, if not earlier, the term *holistic health* began to appear more frequently. Today it has become almost a "dirty" word for some allopathic doctors of medicine. To me it is a profoundly sensible concept, although not readily translated into practice by any one individual healer or practitioner, since it deals with three dimensions: physical, mental, and spiritual. Most practitioners tend to be specialists in one of these three areas: a physician for the physical; a psychiatrist, psychologist or other type of mental-health counselor for the psyche; and a clergyman or spiritual advisor for the soul.

Bringing all three dimensions together simultaneously to elicit true wholeness, healthiness, or holiness is not easy. The realms of mind and body alone are so badly split that there are only small successes in understanding and treating the mind/body unity, as in psychosomatic illnesses, and stress disorders. In psychiatry itself there is scarcely any viable bridging between psychology and religion, or spirituality. The original meaning of the Greek word, *psyche*, was "soul."

Macrobiotics in its most complete definition and practice is truly holistic. I find it too easy to forget this when I speak to my friends or family about macrobiotics, as though it were only a matter of what I eat, or how to cook *azuki* beans or *arame* sea vegetable. The way of life according to the order of the universe is what shapes the nutritional guidelines, and the methods of alternative medicine, as well as other recommendations. It is a psychology, a physical regimen, and a spiritual practice, none of which contradicts or is antagonistic to traditional values. It fits the New Testament message of "having life, and having it more abundantly."

In keeping with the principles of Oriental philosophy, macrobiotics, and some Western views of humankind, we all live amidst paradoxes, polarities, opposites, and complementarities. I am both an enthusiast for macrobiotics and a skeptic. I want scientific support for it. I see some areas of incomplete explanation and contradiction. At the same time I obviously cannot wait ten or twenty years for full documentation to support my personal practices. My participation in August 1986 at the six-day Macrobiotic Camp, sponsored by the Kushi Institute, gave me enough excitement and encountering with two hundred people to sustain me for the next ten months, even without firm proof. I found myself beginning to drift away from healthful actions in the eleventh and twelfth months.

For me the struggle was greatest in cooking enough varied dishes so that I could avoid repeating the same dish literally ad nauseam, or to a point of slight queasiness.

I also began to experience a subversive devilish sense of "Oh, why bother? I feel great, and I can manage without 'fussing' so much." (My arrogant consciousness didn't consider an obvious point: perhaps I felt so well because I had been reasonably consistent, eating a cup of miso soup daily, a *shiitake* mushroom a day, and a fairly regular amount of grains, beans, vegetables, and some sea vegetables. Also, I had eaten almost no cheese, red meats, eggs, and very little poultry. At one point in the eleventh month I ate some good-quality Vermont cheddar cheese and was startled how salty it tasted. I continued, however, to nibble on it for several days. Despite my enjoyment of it, I had absolutely no interest to buy any more. The same thing happened with some Brie cheese. It tasted irresistibly delicious. I was not about to emulate the nun in Franz Werfel's novel, *The Song of Bernadette*. She placed an exquisitely delicious-looking peach on a plate by her beside, in order to contemplate what sacrifice she could endure by not eating it. Sinners are hungrier than saints. So, I ate the Brie, and over the course of a week I finished it. My wife had assisted me only slightly in consuming it. Again, I did not have any subsequent urge to buy or eat any more.

I am now, some many weeks later, aware that the process of developing a macrobiotic style of eating does take more than a year. So-called "relapses" are a natural and normal part of the process. The exception applies for those who must be on a strict healing diet for clear and immediate survival reasons. The very ambiguity of my medical/surgical conditions made it less clearly an indication for constant strictness.

I backslid in several other ways, eating a few more eggs and poultry than I had for the first ten months. In mid-August of 1987 I again attended the Summer Macrobiotic Conference in Great Barrington, Massachusetts. Perhaps I intuitively knew that I would be re-inspired by the experience to correct the deficiencies and excesses that had been occurring. I certainly hoped for that, since I was not comfortable with my drifting away. The experience proved more than re-inspiring. Meeting many more individuals who had serious and potentially fatal conditions, and who were now clearly recovering or were much healthier than they had been, was deeply moving and exciting. Seeing healthy individuals and families actively following a macrobiotic way of eating and living also supported my renewed intentions to remain macrobiotic. The lectures and workshops were instructive, and frequently mind-boggling. The camaraderie and encountering with other participants, from age three to eighty, was soul-soothing.

At this time (October, 1987) I am more committed to maintaining a macrobiotic lifestyle for the next forty years. I am prepared to share my knowledge and experience with those patients I encounter in my practice who wish to learn about macrobiotics. I am giving consideration to preparing more fully for this by taking formal training, in order to utilize it within my practice.

There is no local center in my home area. I plan to support the development of a macrobiotic center, and share the value and pleasure of my macrobiotic experience. "The possibilities are endless" is written on a button my wife wears on her shirt.

During the recent Macrobiotic Conference I underwent my first shiatsu massage. It was given by a director of a midwest macrobiotic center, who also spoke at the conference. I experienced myself afterwards as having gotten both my body and mind straightened out, with more energy unblocked and flowing, sensorily and cognitively. I felt myself standing taller and ready to return home better grounded, on earth, and in macrobiotics.

It is now a month since returning home. I finally discovered a more palatable way to cook and enjoy kale. I am also more liberal in using miso, trying several varieties, such as chick-pea and mellow white, as well as the more actively healing barley miso. I am managing to feel less guilty with occasional deviations, and also not feeling guilty for *not* feeling guilty. I accept the responsibility for any consequences, if I drift too much. My body will inform me. My goal, however, is to rationalize less and deviate less, within a framework that avoids rigidity. I can see that excessive rigidity or strictness can lead to abandonment, and this I wish to avoid. Since harmony and balance are constantly to be sought, this applies to the practice of macrobiotics as well.

My cholesterol level was 270 at the age of thirty-six (1971). My internist, a cardiologist, said nothing in those days, since it was considered "within normal limits." A year ago it was 238. After a few months of macrobiotic eating it was down to 213. A few weeks ago I had the satisfaction of knowing I had gotten below 200, to 199. A modest accomplishment, but nonetheless it felt highly rewarding, and a distinct reinforcement to keep on with my program for myself. Such concrete rewards help support staying with the new approach to health and possible longevity.

I recently attended the eighth annual Maine Healing Arts Festival in Freedom, Maine. About 270 persons attended the three-day conference. Some of us, about 50, attended the workshop on firewalking. Although I had not intended to do other than watch this slightly mysterious, anxiety-provoking, and intriguing procedure, I decided to participate. About 30 of us did in fact walk the ten feet across a bed of burning coals. About a cord of oak burned for two hours to the bed of coals that were walked on. The actual physical experience is simple and not at all dangerous, so long as one follows instructions, pays attention, and neither stands still nor runs. The mind, however, tends to be boggled and surprised. One consequence of the experience is the ability to affirm that one is capable of doing anything one chooses to do. I choose to follow a macrobiotic way of life.

If I succeed in living to one hundred, I prefer not to be like the gentleman of 102 who said," If I knew I was going to live so long, I would have taken better care of myself." It is no joke living a long life if the quality of that life is only a barely tolerable existence. Then it is a minor achievement at best. In recent years there has been an emphasis on the extension of life. Statistics are quite explicit about the increasing percentage of the population that will be over sixty-five and eight-five in the years 2000 and 2020. There needs to be equal interest in how to maintain

ood, comfortable health as well. I suspect that this is an area in
which macrobiotics can be very useful, if started early enough
in life. There are already encouraging signs, as well as alarms.
Children's cholesterol levels are being scrutinized more carefully
and there is already greater awareness of how to feed children
so they can not only achieve longevity, but also experience pleasure in being healthy adults and oldsters.

Pogo has already given us a major clue, when he stated some
years ago, "We have met the enemy, and they are us."

Diet—The Best Medicine

David Dodson, M.D.

Macrobiotics, it seems, was a destiny for me. My first exposure to macrobiotics came in 1970. I was a teenager, and my cousin Stan Street had personally experienced the healing power of macrobiotics. Stan was a mentor for me, and I was very impressed by what he told me, but we lived 3,000 miles apart at the time and I was not to get involved with macrobiotics myself for some time.

In 1971, my family moved to Paris. As fate would have it, I happened to make friends there with a group of people who were practicing macrobiotics. Remembering my cousin's advice that learning about macrobiotics would be very valuable to me, I read my French friends' books and enjoyed the wholesome nutritious food they prepared.

The following year my family returned to Ottawa, Canada, where we had lived since 1957. Many of my old high school friends had moved away, and I wound up with a new circle of friends. Again, quite coincidentally, my new friends were macrobiotic —I had not sought out macrobiotic people, I just did not seem to be able to avoid them!

Coming from a family of scientists, and having a natural aptitude for math and science, I decided to study medicine. Within a few weeks of beginning medical school in September 1975, Dr. Dennis Burkitt gave a lecture entitled "Lessons From Africa For Diseases In Ottawa." The lecture was given in the evening and all members of the Ottawa medical community were invited. Two things that evening were notable: first, that only one of my classmates came, and second, I probably learned more useful information that evening than in the next four years of medical school! Dr. Burkitt is an extremely witty gentleman, and I am sure that the assembled professors and practitioners of medicine had rarely if ever been treated to such an amusing, not to mention informative session.

Dr. Burkitt's thesis, based on his experience as a surgeon in central Africa for over twenty years, is that most of the diseases prevalent in industrialized countries result from the modern diet, in particular from the milling of grains, the result being removal of fiber from the diet. This of course, was very exciting to me. In effect, one of the leading figures in the medical world (that was how Dr. Burkitt was introduced that evening) had given powerful validation to the macrobiotic approach.

I thus started my medical studies on a high note, but unfortunately, many years were to pass before I was to experience this sort of intellectual excitement in medicine again. Most doctors continued—and I am afraid, still continue—to remain horribly ignorant of the connection between diet and health. In fact, the medical profession is so unconcerned with nutrition that I found myself wondering what to do with my medical training. It did not occur to me that I might specialize in nutrition because I never encountered a single doctor in seven years of training who had more than a superficial interest in what their patients ate.

Yet as I studied medicine I became more and more convinced that science verifies the wisdom of macrobiotics. About five years after I had the fortune of hearing Dr. Burkitt speak, I was again privileged to hear one of the "giants" in medicine: Dr. William Castelli, director of the prestigious Framingham Heart Study. Dr. Castelli's lecture had the provocative title "Is Atherosclerosis Reversible?" and the amazing answer to his rhetorical question was yes. Dr. Castelli pointed out that *atherosclerosis* or the buildup of cholesterol-containing plaques in the arteries which leads to strokes, heart attacks, and other serious conditions, is present only among people who eat high-fat diets based on large amounts of animal foods. Dr. Castelli remarked that after six months on a hospital diet, monkeys' arteries become so clogged that they need amputations due to lack of circulation in the legs. Dr. Castelli has demonstrated reversal of atherosclerosis in monkeys, and evidence is now accumulating that shows that humans can also reverse the process of atherosclerotic narrowing of the arteries. Dr. Castelli has examined the blood of macrobiotic people and found them to have cholesterol levels so low that not only would heart attacks be virtually impossible, but those who had already developed atherosclerosis would be likely to reverse it—in other words, unclog their arteries.

Upon finishing medical school in Canada, I returned to the United States, and trained in internal medicine at Harvard. Again, I just happened to meet a macrobiotic person who was also studying at Harvard. That person had been practicing macrobiotics since his birth—Lawrence Haruo Kushi, Michio's son.

I finally decided to formally study nutrition. There are sixteen hospitals in the United States that train M.D.s in nutrition, and fortunately for me, three of them are in Boston. I decided to do a fellowship in clinical nutrition at Boston University, as B. U. was the center of ongoing research into various aspects of macrobiotics. Every year, over 10,000 new doctors graduate from medical schools in the United States. Of those, up to 36 go on to train in nutrition. I had finally found my niche in medicine by joining that elite corps!

The symbol of yin and yang shows the seed of yin within the yang and vice versa. This symbolizes my experience as a medical scientist: the more I learn scientifically about medicine and nutrition, the more the beauty and power of macrobiotics to promote health becomes apparent to me. Thus science has no conflict with macrobiotics. Quite the contrary, science complements the Oriental approach, a marriage which I feel was made in heaven. Obviously, my views are not shared by all scientists, many of whom have had very closed minds concerning macrobiotics. One is reminded of the often quoted words of the famous physicist Max Planck that," An important scientific innovation rarely makes its way by gradually winning over and converting its opponents: it rarely happens that Saul becomes Paul. What does happen is that its opponents gradually die out and that the growing generation is familiarized with the idea from the beginning."

It is said that an ounce of prevention is worth a pound of cure, though my observations lead me to believe that an ounce of prevention may actually be worth a few tons of cure. The amount of prevention that macrobiotics could accomplish is truly staggering. It is very exciting for me as a physician to be involved with macrobiotics, and I will be forever grateful for the opportunity this represents. The following examples will, I hope, help to show why I feel this way.

On May 8, 1986 the *New England Journal of Medicine* published an article entitled "Progress Against Cancer?" which pointed out that in spite of the war on cancer, age adjusted incidence and mortality rates for cancer have been increasing steadily for over twenty-five years. Though dramatic progress has been made against a few rare forms of cancer, these types of cancers only constitute about 2 percent of all cancers. For the great majority of common cancers little or no progress has been made in decades. The authors suggested that research should be shifted away from trying to find the cure that is always "just out of reach" towards research aimed at preventing cancer from developing in the first place. Similar views were expressed in the *Scientific American** by Dr. John Cairns who stated that most forms of cancer are preventable. Dr. Cairns also pointed out that all of mankind's previous scourges such as scurvey, pellagra, smallpox, plague, tuberculosis, typhus, polio, and so on, were conquered through prevention, not cure, and thus the "war on cancer," in searching for a cure, ignores the history of how all prior public health problems have been solved.

This is not to say that macrobiotics cannot help those people who have already developed cancer. Certainly the stories of Anthony Sattilaro, M.D., Elaine Nussbaum, and others who recovered from cancer through macrobiotics have inspired countless cancer patients to begin the macrobiotic way of life. Though as yet statistics are not available on the success rate of macrobiotics in cancer, research is currently in progress at Boston University to determine this. My own experience has showed me that even in advanced cases of cancer, macrobiotics certainly improves the quality of life quite apart from any effect on the duration of life.

In terms of preventing cancer though, science has much more to say. It is now generally agreed among experts that the great majority of cancers—up to 90 percent—are preventable. An edi-

---

* Cairns, J., "The Treatment of Diseases and the War Against Cancer." *Scientific American* vol. 253 pp. 51–9, Nov. 1985.

orial by Drs. Gori and Wynder which appeared in the *Journal of the National Cancer Institute* in 1974 stated that more cancers could be prevented through dietary improvements than through any other means including the elimination of smoking. Dietary recommendations were made in 1982 by the National Research Council's Diet, Nutrition, and Cancer Panel. They recommended less fat consumption, more whole grains, and more fresh vegetables and fruits. These same recommendations have been made by macrobiotic people for decades! Many other organizations including the American Heart Association, the U.S. Senate Select Committee on Nutrition and Human Needs, and the U.S. Department of Agriculture have also jumped on the bandwagon with similar recommendations.

In 1981 the Center for Disease Control discovered a dreadful new sexually transmitted disease. This new disease is perhaps more frightening than any science-fiction author could have imagined. There have been over 40,000 cases in the United States as of this writing and the incidence of new cases is increasing exponentially. Most of the victims of this nightmare called AIDS are already dead, and current medical thinking is that all of those still alive will die unless some breakthrough in the treatment of this tragic condition is found.

It is estimated that as many as two million Americans may already be infected with the *Human Immunodeficiency Virus*, or HIV, that is believed to cause AIDS. It is not known how many of those infected with HIV will develop AIDS, though it is currently estimated that perhaps as many as one-third of infected individuals will develop either AIDS or the AIDS related complex of symptoms known as ARC. An obvious question to ask is what distinguishes the majority of people infected with HIV who have so far remained well from those who have developed AIDS or ARC? In thinking about this question, I am struck by the fact that all of the immunologic abnormalities seen in AIDS can also be seen in malnutrition. Does diet interact with the HIV virus to produce AIDS? Such nutrients as zinc, iron, selenium, folic acid, and fat are all known to effect immune function, so such an interaction is indeed probable.

In 1984 Michio Kushi began working with a group of men

with AIDS who have been practicing macrobiotics. Blood samples from these men have been sent to Boston University where research is being conducted in the Department of Microbiology. Analysis of these samples has indeed shown improvement in the blood of these men. This data was presented at the Second International Conference on AIDS held in Paris in July 1986. I have been working with several colleagues in Boston to pursue these preliminary but promising results.

A precursor to many of the chronic diseases that plague our society is obesity. Diabetes, high blood pressure, arthritis, many forms of cancer are just a few examples of diseases associated with obesity. Macrobiotics is definitely the ultimate weight-control diet. Overweight macrobiotic people are rare, and gross obesity is virtually non-existent on the macrobiotic diet. Best of all, one who learns to enjoy eating macrobiotically never has to count their calories, but can enjoy three good meals daily complete with second helpings and dessert! As long as one eats macrobiotically, the weight will stay off, and this is of key importance because when people go on and off the usual sort of weight-loss diets, the weight also goes on and off. This subject, along with a detailed discussion of modern nutrition science is discussed in my book (co-authored with my wife Marianne) *Eat More, Weigh Less*.

Marianne has always insisted on buying the best-quality organic produce available. Her attitude is that it would be foolish to try to save money by buying inferior-quality food which may result in reducing the quality—possibly even the quantity— of our lives through sickness.

A recent ruling by the Food and Drug Administration (FDA) may constitute one of the worse threats yet to our food supply. On April 18, 1986 the FDA approved the use of ionizing radiation to preserve food. Because of the seriousness of this issue to anyone concerned with quality food and health, I will discuss food irradiation at some length. Joseph Roberts of the Canadian Coalition to Stop Food Irradiation says that food irradiation is such a questionable affair it ought to be referred to as irradiation of foods, or IF. For convenience, I will use Joseph's abbreviation.

The concept of IF has been around for many decades and the U.S government has spent over 80 million dollars on research attempting to demonstrate the safety of IF. Nevertheless, many people are convinced—FDA approval notwithstanding—that IF is unsafe, unwise, and just plain stupid.

Ionizing radiation is a type of energy that disrupts the chemical bonds between the atoms that are joined together to form the molecules that our bodies, our food, and the entire physical world are made of. This results in the formation of new chemicals, including ions (hence the term ionizing radiation) and free radicals. These ions and free radicals in turn cause further alteration in the chemical structure of the food, bacteria, or whatever else is being irradiated.

In practical terms, this means that insects that are eating harvested grains can be killed by irradiating the grain, and certain harmful organisms in the food supply (e.g. trichinella in pork, or salmonella in chicken) can be killed by irradiating the food in question. It has also been suggested that by killing bacteria that cause spoilage, the shelf life of food can be prolonged. Proponents of IF even suggest that IF would be useful to combat world hunger. They also claim that IF will reduce the need for chemicals used in food production.

When looked at carefully, these arguments in favor of IF lose all merit. In responses to the above examples:

• Insects will eat grain whether or not it has been irradiated. More appropriate technologies, such as storing grains in carbon dioxide gas (which all plants inhale, but all animal life including insects exhale) are available to reduce post-harvest loss to insects.
• There were 43 cases of trichinosis in all of the United States in an entire year. All of these cases could have been prevented by properly cooking the pork, as cooking kills the trichinella parasite. To irradiate everyone's pork due to this rare and easily prevented disease is patentedly absurd.
• Likewise, salmonella germs are also killed by proper cooking. More importantly, salmonella represents fecal contamination, which routinely occurs in the factories that mechanically slaughter chickens by the thousands every day. This mechanical process

results in very high rates of contamination. Clearly, the ideal response to the problem would be to get the chicken producers to clean up their act, not to take contaminated chicken and irradiate them. After all, irradiated fecal material may be sterilized, but it is still fecal material and consumers should not have to eat it. Again, IF is not the answer!

• The claim that IF is needed to combat world hunger is a particularly cynical and dishonest one. In fact, plenty of food is produced to feed all the world's hungry people. An editorial on the subject of the world food glut appeared in *Science*, the official journal of the American Association for the Advancement of Science, on April 3, 1987, and the subject was also discussed at length in the *New York Times* on September 9, 1986, on page 19. In fact, hunger occurs for political reasons and NOT due to lack of food in the world. The United States government has stockpiles in excess of *five billions pounds* of milk, cheese, and butter bought to support dairy prices and furthermore pays vast sums of money to support the tobacco-growing industry. Let the government feed hungry people instead of vast warehouses and let the government stop helping farmers grow poisonous tobacco and instead help them grow food before they tell us we need IF to feed the world's hungry people. The most appropriate technology to improve the food supply in developing countries is refrigeration, not food irradiation.

There is evidence that IF may result in use of more, not less chemicals in food processing. One example is in Japan where Hokkaido potatoes have been irradiated for several years. This vegetable requires complex treatment which includes additional chemicals to make it suitable for irradiation. Another example is the irradiation of meat, which requires treatment with tripolyphosphate to stablize the fats. *Tripolyphosphate* is a solvent compound useful for removing grime from walls and floors. Even if I did eat meat, I surely would not want to consume meat that had been subjected to such treatment.

A considerable body of scientific evidence has shown that the consumption of irradiated foods is unsafe, and in particular, that such foods have *radiomimetic properties*—that is, eating irradiated foods may mimic the effects of actual exposure to radiation. I will briefly discuss some of the evidence for this.

Experiments done over twenty years ago looked at the effect of growing human white blood cells in the presence of nutrient solutions that had been irradiated. It is important to understand that these solutions were not radioactive, nor is irradiated food. Nevertheless, the white blood cells that were fed the irradiated solutions developed chromosomal damage similar to that which would be caused by exposing the cells themselves to radiation. Such damage did not occur when cells were grown in identical solutions that had not been irradiated.

In the mid-seventies, freshly irradiated wheat was fed to a group of children in India and a control group of children were fed a diet that was identical except that it had not been irradiated. The children fed the irradiated food developed an abnormality of their blood cells called *polyploidy*, meaning the appearance of extra chromosomes (chromosomes contain genetic information in the form of DNA). The children eating the normal diet had no such problem. The experiment was repeated using wheat that had been stored for twelve weeks after irradiation. This time polyploidy again occurred, but not as rapidly or as severely as when it was fed to the children within two to three weeks of having been irradiated. Similar experiments with similar results have been carried out using rats, mice, hamsters, and monkeys, instead of children. Although the polyploidy gradually disappeared when the children went back to eating normal food and the significance of polyploidy is unknown, polyploidy can be associated with cancer and these experiments remain strong evidence against the safety of eating irradiated foods.

IF results in the formation of new chemicals in the irradiated foods. As such, it can only reasonably be considered an additive as far as FDA (Food and Drug Administration) regulations are concerned. Industry, however, wants it considered as a process such as canning or freezing rather than an additive so that they will not be subject to the strict regulations governing food additives. The FDA has sided with industry, agreeing to consider IF as a process.

Nevertheless, by their own estimation, the FDA assumes that

IF will result in the addition of about 3 ppm (parts per million) of new chemicals known as *unique radiolytic products,* or URPs. This may not sound like much, but at that rate, if a person ate a diet that consisted of 100 percent irradiated foods from the time of their birth, by the age of fifty, the total amount of URPs consumed would amount to about one ounce. That by no means is a trival amount in any sane person's estimation, but it apparently is considered trivial and not worth worrying about as far as the FDA is concerned.

Another way to place the figure of 3 ppm into perspective is that aflatoxin is known to produce cancer in concentrations as low as *one part per billion.* Thus by the FDAs own estimates, URPs will be present in irradiated food in amounts 2,000 times higher than that which causes cancer in the case of aflatoxins. What if URPs turn out to be as toxic as aflatoxins—or even more toxic?

The point is that before IF can be promoted as a safe technology, it is absolutely essential that the URPs be carefully tested. The FDA is handing out the line that this cannot be done. That is not true; URPs could be extracted, concentrated, and tested. However, if the FDA were correct in saying that testing URPs is impossible, then I would submit that that in itself would constitute a strong argument against IF.

In addition to the above objections to IF, many people feel that its environmental impact would also be unhealthy, to say the least. The proponents of IF envision IF as providing a use for spent fuel from nuclear reactors, both commercial and military. Such spent fuel is the major problem associated with nuclear reactors as it remains highly radioactive. Plans call for the reprocessing of this spent fuel to extract isotopes such as cesium 137 which could be used for IF.

Some people actually regard IF as a mere excuse to build such a reprocessing plant which would also be able to extract weapons-grade plutonium from spent fuel. The reason this would be an attractive approach for the military is that the machines which currently produce plutonium for bombs are old and in need of replacement, but the replacement costs are so high as to be virtually prohibitive (see the *New York Times,* March 13, 1987, page A 15). Enter IF—providing a market for reprocessed spent nuclear fuel, providing the military with a solution for its plutonium procurement problem, and establishing a new nuclear-food industry. Though this may sound like just another paranoid conspiracy theory, it explains a number of irregularities: for one, the military has been the prime researcher and the government the prime promoter of IF. Normally the promoter of a new food process or chemical additive applies to the FDA for approval and is subject to long, careful, and detailed studies before the approval is granted. In this case, it is the FDA itself that is pushing the approval of IF, and needless to say, they have not followed their usual rigorous procedures to prove its safety.

Regardless of why the government is pushing IF, plans call for building a reprocessing plant and shipping huge amounts of radioactive wastes to this plant and then shipping huge amounts of radioactive cesium 137 to the food irradiation plants, which will be all over the country if proponents of IF have their way. Because accidents do indeed happen, shipping such tremendous amounts of radioactive materials virtually guarantees that there will eventually be a catastrophic spill of deadly radioactive materials.

Fortunately, some politicians have understood the madness of IF and its potential to harm the people. California representative Douglas Bosco has introduced bill # HR956 which calls for a moratorium on IF pending adequate studies, and a companion bill, # S461 has been introduced by Maine Senator George Mitchell. I urge the reader to contact his or her congressmen and ask them to support these bills. Further information on the subject can be obtained from the excellent San Francisco organization National Coalition to Stop Food Irradiation.

Good food that is natural and not irradiated is the best preventive medicine; poor diet contributes to much if not most of the chronic illness that constitutes the major threat to health throughout the developed world. In this essay I have tried to discuss briefly why I feel that modern nutritional science is saying the same thing that macrobiotics is saying: if you take responsibility for your health and eat well, you can expect to live not only longer but to live better, free of the chronic aliments that are now epidemic in our society. It is a great privilege for me as a physician to have such a powerful tool as macrobiotics to share with my patients, and I cannot recommend it too strongly for those who wish to enjoy good health.

On My Awakening to the Macrobiotic Way

Stephen Harnish, M.D.

The first patient I examined as a beginning medical student at the University of New Mexico was a psychotic young man on a medical ward. He had eaten *Drano* and burned his esophagus right out of his chest. He could no longer eat food. Instead a tube went directly to his stomach with specially prepared nutrients. This did not seem to affect this young man's delusions which included his belief he was God. I can just imagine how wide-eyed I must have returned to the upperclassman when I reported my examination of this psychotic, self-destructive enigma who thought himself divine.

As I plunged into my description of the case the older medical students chuckled at my awe and attempted to guide my thinking in a clinical pattern: chief complaint, history of present illness, past history, family history, and so on. I remember feeling tricked; a psychiatric patient on a medical ward who had been suicidal and I was supposed to remain calm and clinical? I wonder if the fact that I am now a psychiatrist, despite my initial inclination to be a family doctor, had anything to do with the impact this first patient had on me as a student barely two weeks into the four-year program.

As the years went on, I too became calm and clinical, probably as a self-defense while medical school proceeded to steal my innocence and burden my psyche with every imaginable disease, infection, trauma, tumor, birth defect or mental disorder. Somehow, I left medical school with the impression that the question "why?" was either irrelevant or impossible to answer. "Because" seemed the only answer. Why did the intern's young wife die shortly after I, as a medical student, examined her for her final course of chemotherapy? Because God made it that way? Because she wasn't one of the lucky ones? The unspoken attitude was "don't bother with why, concentrate on how (to fix it), what (is it), when (did it start), who (else in the family has had it before). This all served me well at the time, I thought. I learned the latest techniques to discover, diagnose, evaluate, plapate, osculate, treat and then retreat if necessary without ever answering why do they have this condition to begin with, why don't we know more about the etiology of illness, why wasn't I taught more about nutrition?

During my psychiatric residency at the Dartmouth Medical School I continued to ponder why questions. These had to do with the suffering of people with mental disorders, the urges they have to end their lives, the mysteries of their psychosis, the devastation of their lives ruined by drug abuse and even crime. Why do people behave as they do, I wondered? Why does some people's behavior seem so out of control?

I learned about the neurobiochemical basis of mental illness. That was fine and the theories seemed to make sense. They even justified the chemotherapy needed to correct the chemically based psychopathology, but why did the person's biochemistry malfunction to begin with? Was it a genetic predisposition or even an inherited defect? Was it a reaction to others? Was it a person giving up and needing others to assume care of them?

I began working on a practical theory that might explain, at least in a conceptual way, how behavior for any one individual may be determined. It seemed, as I worked with many psychotherapy patients, that much of their emotional pain, be it anxiety, depression, or even psychosis, came from their feeling stuck. They were stuck in a bad job or stuck in a painful relationship or stuck on ruminations about childhood. In fact there seemed to be hundreds of stuck situations they would describe to me during the many hours I would work with them in psychotherapy. A common theme emerged about this stuckness—the individuals felt it was out of their control. They knew they should do this or ought to do that or even must change, but they could not, they were stuck.

As I revealed their trap to the patient and as they worked their way out of their suffering, I noticed they moved from a psychological position of "I must," to "I need to," and finally to "I want to." It seemed amazing that the same issue as a "must" would cause great emotional distress, but as a "need," less distress, and as a "want," none at all, maybe even pleasure. For example, a young mother caring for an infant child while still holding down a full-time job, experienced great emotional distress because she felt totally trapped and stuck. She felt she must provide loving child care and efficient work performance no matter what. She believed she should be kind and gentle with the child. She believed she ought to be productive and alert at work. As she began to fail her own shoulds and oughts, her feeling that she must do better intensified, as did her sense of inadequacy and her rage at her situation, at her trap. Finally she came to me for help when one morning, while trying to patiently feed breakfast to the baby who sat in the high chair, she grabbed a frying pan and smashed it through the wall in utter frustration. Her behavior was out of her control, her life felt out of her control, she sensed she did everything for others, nothing for herself. She feared she would crack-up, she could not sleep, she had trouble concentrating, and she began to fear she might hurt herself or, God forbid, the baby.

As I began her treatment I knew her symptoms pointed to depression, her neurochemistry may be malfunctioning, her genetic predisposition for mental illness may have been triggered by her building emotional pressure, she may need an antidepressant medication and a pill to help her sleep, but she also had to get unstuck! Medication provided some initial symptomatic relief. Knowing she had the right, under the circumstances, to feel like she might have a breakdown helped, but not until she was able to untie the knots of her trap was she able to regain her health and her sense of control of her life. As I observed the process of her psychotherapy we were able to move her approach to her life from feeling motivated to appease the musts in her life and change them to needs, and finally to a desire to want to do those things which initially had felt so burdensome. We knew she had regained her health when she no longer needed medication and when she wanted (for the most part, give or take a bad day) to get up to feed the baby, she wanted to go to work, she wanted to be alive.

As I pondered this phenomenon with this patient and many other similar cases, I began to develop a theory of motivation of behavior. It seemed to begin to answer my why questions about behavior. When a person feels compelled to perform, their behavior willed by others and not themselves, they feel stuck and trapped as if their life is out of their control. When the motivation feels more like a need, self-control begins to play a larger role in motivating their behavior and it seems more comfortable. When the motivation is purely a want, the feeling of the self being in control is complete and stress, traps, stuckness, or eventual mental illness seems far away. As a simple example, I would ask my patients to consider how they felt in response to the following three short statements: I must eat; I need to eat; I want to eat. In the first case the patients agreed there was considerable stress, as if the person was starving. In the second case the patients understood there seemed to be some choice, "I know I should eat but I have some time and I'll do it when I can." Here, some self-control emerges. In the final I want to eat, the patients expressed a vision of pleasure and desire, of self-control with no trap involved.

Fig. 2 Trilogy of Desire

A continuum showing the relationships of self-control and other control, divided into sections labled Want, Need and Must.

		WANT	NEED	MUST	
Self-Control	100%		50%		0% Self-Control
Other Control	0%		50%		100% Other Control
		WANT	NEED	MUST	

The theory I called the *Trilogy of Desire* is based on the three positions of behavior motivation of an individual; must, need, and want. This was all well and good for some patients but why others behaved as they did still confounded me, such as the psychotic killer I faced one night at the state hospital while I was on-call as part of my residency. The patient knew the process better than me: cause a ruckus, don't calm down when the nurse comes, demand to see the doctor on-call and then give him hell. "It's these voices, doc, you are a doctor, aren't you? Are you sure you're out of college, how old are you anyhow? The voices, yes they torment me, they call me names, they tell me to kill myself, just like they told me to kill my mother, I'm scared, 'cause I killed her, you gotta help me doc." He popped the top of another in a series of colas and stared at me defiantly. When I mentioned a medicine, he either had it, hated it, or was already on it. "Why am I like this doc?" he would ask as he took another swig of cola. "Sometimes I get wired and I gotta hurt myself to calm down." He showed me the scars up his left forearm from years of slashing. "Gimme something to knock me out" he would plead. I wondered if he just liked to make the residents squirm. Too bad I didn't ask him about the cola, or the rest of his diet, or of his spiritual life. Why must he behave like this? How could I help him want to be healthy?

Some years later, I was medical director of that state hospital. I felt pressured to know all the answers but there seemed to be many more questions than answers, especially concerning why these poor suffering souls were confined to a state hospital with uremitting or recurring psychosis. The Trilogy of Desire seemed lost in the past. During my tenure as medical director I never went to the kitchen and asked about the diet we provided, or asked the patients how they ate when they went home or what snacks they bought at the canteen. Instead I was concerned because patients would, at will, refuse any and all treatment, whether they were competent to make a decision or not. I was greatly distressed that many of the severely psychotic patients on our crowded wards were showing no improvement. Many, from the date of their emergency commitment would adamantly refuse any and all therapeutic intervention including individual therapy, group therapy, and especially medication. I agonized over these cases because no improvement occurred, longer commitments resulted, an expensive hospital bed was used for no good reason

I thought, and the patient's personal psychic torment continued. This situation finally came to the public's attention in a series of articles in the state hospital's local newspaper, *The Concord Monitor*. In one article by David Olinger entitled, "Dispensing Drugs: A Delicate Problem,"[1] he wrote:

"He had seen her, 'a very delicate young woman,' scratching at the screen covering the hospital window. She had imagined that her mother was standing just outside the building.

"She was looking out the window, crying, 'Mother, come get me, Why aren't you coming to get me?' She stayed up all night doing that.

"'Now she's not dangerous, but she sure is suffering. Honestly, it breaks my heart to see that suffering going on while my hands are tied.'

"Dr. Stephen Harnish warmed to the theme. Twenty of the 74 involuntarily committed patients at New Hampshire Hospital had refused to sign authorizations for treatment; nine of 59 patients in the forensic unit were also refusing medicine.

"The court-committed patients 'are angry as hell,' he said. 'They didn't want to be here. They impede other people from getting well. They hurt staff, they hurt other patients. And they take up most of the time—it's the squeaky wheel syndrome.'

"'Even if they've been committed, we're still not allowed to treat them. Then, only if I declare an emergency can I medicate.'

"'The psychiatric staff has been intimidated by the courts. They don't want to get stuck. They don't want a suit brought against them. The courts are saying, 'Here's a car, fix it. And by the way, you can't have your tool box. Only if you think the car's going to self-destruct can you use a screw driver, and then only for a little while.'

"'One of our most serious problems here is our lack of ability to treat people who are very, very sick and suffering.'"

In desperation I won a seat in the state legislature, resigned as medical director, sat on the legislative health and welfare committee, introduced legislation to facilitate treatment for committed patients but never asked my state program about nutrition or diet and I never asked the Trilogy of Desire to help me with the why of all this.

Then my life changed. I met Marsha, my future wife, who worked on the legislative staff. As our relationship developed I found myself in awe of her knowledge of human nature and health. She knew how to deal with why. Because we do it to ourselves she taught me. I finally learned this lesson in a dramatic way. When I met her father, my future father-in-law, he was on his death bed. He was dying of cancer. It seemed I had barely asked him for his daughter's hand when a few days later he died. Marsha gently told me of the visits for chemotherapy when she had accompanied her father to the hospital, of her search through the library for any clue to what might help, of her discovery of macrobiotics, and her desire to help her father with diet. But he died too soon. Later, after we married, Marsha and I slowly pursued our search for a healthy lifestyle. We began to eat more carefully, we bought the *American Heart Association Cookbook*.[2] The Association's dietary recommendations, referred to as a fat-controlled diet designed to reduce blood lipids (fat)—can be summarized as follows:

1. A caloric intake adjusted to achieve and maintain ideal body weight.
2. A reduction in total fat calories achieved by a substantial reduction in dietary saturated fatty acids. The total fat in the diet should comprise no more than 30 to 35 percent of total calories. The level of saturated fatty acids should be decreased to less than 10 percent of total calories.
3. A substantial reduction in dietary cholesterol to less than 300 mgs. daily.
4. Dietary carbohydrate primarily derived from vegetables, fruits, whole grain and enriched breads and cereals.
5. Avoidance of excessive sodium in the diet.

According to the Association:
"Effectiveness of the diet in lowering serum cholesterol and consequently reducing one of the risks of heart attack is dependent upon proper choice of foods relative to their fat and cholesterol content. A basic principle to keep in mind is that food products from animal sources contain cholesterol; food products from land animals also have saturated fat; and food products from

aquatic animals contain primarily polyunsaturated fat. Polyunsaturated, monounsaturated, and saturated are just so many words—until their part in the total food plan is clear. Most foods contain all three types of fat but in varying amounts. Foods are classified according to their predominant fat content.

"Polyunsaturated fats are those that tend to help the body get rid of newly formed cholesterol and thereby keep the blood cholesterol level down and reduce cholesterol deposition in the arterial walls. Some of the world's greatest cooking oils—safflower, soybean, corn, cottonseed, and sesame seed—have this property. As liquid vegetable oils, they have the highest concentrations of polyunsaturated fatty acids and no cholesterol.

"Olive and peanut oils are also liquid and of vegetable origin, but they contain largely monounsaturated fatty acids and not the beneficial polyunsaturated ones. They do not contain cholesterol, but neither do they have a cholesterol-lowering action.

"On the other hand, foods high in saturated fats tend to elevate the cholesterol concentration in the blood and frequently contain cholesterol itself. These foods include meat, lard, butter and whole-milk dairy products, all high in fats of animal origin."

Because we both seemed to suffer from migraine headaches, we began to study the dietary recommendations from *The Migraine Prevention Cookbook* by Josie D. Wentworth.[3] Important issues we learned and began to incorporate into our lives included information that "research does show that certain things will trigger migraine in susceptible individuals." The list of triggers is extensive, but when these are examined carefully they can be combined within six major categories:

1. Food sensitivity/allergy
2. Hypoglycemia/low blood sugar
3. Tension and stress
4. Water retention
5. Depression
6. Menstruation and the contraceptive pill

It is unfortunate that a large number of sufferers are quite unaware of all the things that can trigger their migraines. For a long time doctors have told their patients that migraine is caused by stress and tension; and so many sufferers have always thought their attacks to be a result of emotional stress, without ever becoming aware of the real culprit.

According to Wentworth:
"Foods that appear to precipitate migraine are those that contain vaso-active amines. Tyramine, phenylethylamine, histamine, isoamylamine, octopamine, synephrine, and 5-hydroxtryptamine are just some of the offending aimes."

Some of the foods containing vaso-active amines are cheese, chocolate, citrus fruits and alcohol. The book discusses these foods in detail as well as provides sample recipies. Wentworth adds: "Another thing to remember about triggers is that their effect is cumulative. You may be able to cope with one trigger, but add two or three together and it is unlikely that you will escape an attack. For example, a person who has had a stressful day, has skipped lunch, is ravenously hungry, and so decides to eat a bar of chocolate is far more likely to develop a migraine than the same person on a restful day, when he or she has eaten regularly and decides to have a chocolate at the end of an enjoyable meal."

We began to watch our diet even more carefully and we eliminated these foods with headache-producing potential. I was curious to observe that diet had become a major area of study and change in our lives. I finally understood how diet was so important after I attended a conference on self-hypnosis presented by the Doctors Spiegel, father and son. In their book *Trance and Treatement—Clinical Uses of Hypnosis*[4] they describe an approach using self-hyponosis for eating disorders. This approach clarified for me what my wife and I seemed to be trying to do—care for our bodies and prevent illness. The Spiegels' approach teaches that through self-hypnosis the patient will practice and learn:

1. For your body overeating is in effect poison. This is just

like the situation with water; you need water to live but too much water will drown you. Similarly, you need food to live but too much of this very same food in effect becomes poison.

2. You cannot live without your body. Your body is the precious physical plant through which you experience life.

3. To the extent that you want to live your life to its fullest, you owe your body this commitment to respect it and protect it. This is your way of acknowledging the fragile, precious nature of your body and at the same time it is your way of seeing yourself as your body's keeper. You are in truth your body's keeper.

When you make this commitment to respect your body, you have within you the power to so radically change your eating and drinking behavior that each eating experience becomes for you an exercise in disciplined respect for your body integrity.

With this all in mind we pushed on to provide a healthier lifestyle for ourselves. I did not run for a second term in the legislature, I took a quiet job as staff psychiatrist at a mental health center. Then Marsha's thyroid condition flared up into an autoimmune form of *thyroiditis*, her immune system was actually attacking and destroying her own thyroid. How, we wondered, could her body do this? Despite our healthy efforts, how could this happen? Her doctor didn't know and offered thyroid pills. Confident we could find better answers we went for a personal interview at the Kushi Institute. There our lives took a dramatic step forward. Through classes and discussion we learned of the need to bring our bodies into harmony with nature through diet, through the macrobiotic way.

Initially the diet was exciting. The flavors and textures were new. The cooking fragrances seemed unusual. Happily we launched into our new diet, keeping careful records of daily meals to assure that we had the right amounts of the food groups. We pressure-cooked our rice, we switched to stainless-steel cookware. We even used a gas camp stove for cooking since our range was electric. I took *sushi* to work for snacks, I used leftovers for lunch. We were mighty pleased with ourselves. Then the novelty wore off and I started noticing a few cravings I had not known of, like for pizza and cake. I tried these again, of course, and my body reacted just as I was told it would, with headaches, diarrhea, and lethargy.

It did not take long for me to realize my body knew something I suspected, my old diet was harmful to me. But the cravings started driving me up the walls. I found myself saying to Marsha, "Do you remember pizza with extra cheese and pepperoni?" or "Whatever happened to your recipe for pound cake with glazed icing?" I began to feel that my diet was out of my control. "Why was I macrobiotic anyhow, I was feeling just fine," I would argue with myself. "I may have had headaches and hay fever, stomach upsets and colds before, which I don't now, but does macrobiotics have anything to do with this?" I felt disgusted. I was trapped. I could always eat out for lunch, but then I wouldn't feel too great for a few days. I thought I must adhere to the diet even though Oreo cookies were so good. I was stuck.

Finally I remembered my Trilogy of Desire (Fig. 2). I realized I was suffering from motivation of the "must" kind. I felt like my behavior was controlled by others. Slowly I worked on my attitude. I tried to put into my motivation all I had learned before from the Heart Association, from the *Migraine Prevention Cookbook* and the self-hypnosis approach of being the protector of my body. I moved mentally to a position of needing to be macrobiotic. At least I had gained the middle portion of the Trilogy of Desire. At least I could own some of the motivation as coming from my own will and desire. With time and effort I remained true to the diet. I dreamed of other foods. I wondered why this was harder than stopping smoking a year earlier and then I knew. I wanted to stop smoking so I did and that was that. I had good reasons, not the least of which was my smokers breath which interfered with my romancing my future wife. So quitting smoking was easy. Now I needed to internalize my desire to remain macrobiotic not for fun or for convenience or even for Marsha, but for myself and my health. This helped push me over the line in the Trilogy of Desire into the want area.

I began to eat macrobiotically because I wanted to; I was relieved, I even found pleasure in my health and my weight (I lost

17 pounds). I no longer ate solely to satisfy my palate but to pursue a lifestyle I knew would provide me with a better life. Thus we were converted, not without some hardship, such as when wanting to eat out. Many a time we would happily be seated at a nice restaurant only to find there really was nothing we could order. We found a few acceptable restaurants within an hour of home but this made the process time consuming—we had to be very desperate to go out. One motivating factor was to find relief from the hours of preparation time. Marsha would begin in the morning and by evening we were set for dinner and the next day's lunch and snack and that was it. Day after day she toiled in the kitchen becoming quick and more efficient but always spending many more hours a day with food preparation than before.

I must admit we became a little "preachy" to our friends and family about our food. "What is that stuff?" they would ask, "it looks like dead worms." We would launch into our description of *hijiki* and the great food value of sea vegetables (not seeweed!). My collegues at work would look over my shoulder at lunch meetings to see what "guru food" I had for that day. Frequently people would ask "Where do you get that stuff anyway?" This too was a problem in rural New Hampshire. We would travel to towns and cities, usually close to an hour away, to natural food stores. Often these speciality stores would have some but not all of our shopping needs. Once a month we would flee to Boston for a Saturday dinner at a macrobiotic restaurant and a "stocking up" grocery shopping. Only occasionally would we ask each other if it was worth all this effort. When we thought of the alternatives, we knew it was. Marsha's condition was improving and within a year her autoimmune system corrected itself and her thyroid size decreased to the smallest size in years.

Along with diet and perhaps because of the diet we found ourselves exploring new avenues of health. Marsha encouraged me to consider meditation, which I did and we began meditating together. The boundaries of my medical curiosity began to expand as well. I found myself exploring environmental illness and the field of clinical ecology. Iris R. Bell, M.D., Ph.D. writes in his book *Clinical Ecology—A New Approach To Environmental Illness*,[5] "the hypothesis is that diverse external stimuli—such as natural inhalants, foods, chemicals, physical factors and psychosocial stresses—can converge on some common pathways in the body early in the genesis of disease. The later divergence in the expression of particular outcomes or illnesses within a population depends upon the inherent tendency of the individual patients towards susceptibility in a particular organ system." This idea brought together in my mind the benefits of the macrobiotic way (not just the diet) and the prevention of illness. I began to look closer at my patients—nearly 1,000 chronically and severely mentally ill people, many previously state-hospital patients, now well enough to attend my outpatient clinic but still taking strong psychotropic medications. I found not only were their diets in chaos but they seemed to put themselves into situations where they experienced many "diverse external stimuli" which would contribute to their illness. These did include "natural inhalants, foods, chemicals, physical factors, and psychosocial stressors." As my eyes opened to these contributions to illness, I realized it was small wonder the medication I prescribed did not do the job I hoped.

The following two case examples illustrate the type of patients I treat and how my new awareness changed the course of their treatment. The first, Judy, is a young woman with a history of severe depression who had been admitted to the state hospital two years ago. She had suffered from poor sleep, tearfulness, trouble concentrating, and suicidal intentions. She was treated at the state hospital with the usual anti-depressant as well as antipsychotic medications. She was discharged to my department fragile and somewhat better—at least she was able to concentrate and sleep, she had no suicidal tendencies. The discharge summary from the hosptial casually mentioned she had been found to have a very low blood sugar and noted she probably suffered from hypoglycemia. No follow up was recommended.

My department supervised a five-hour glucose tolerance test at the local medical center. The results confirmed a hypoglycemic condition. The center counseled her in the traditional hypoglycemic diet which included frequent small meals (5 to 6 per day), the avoidance of sweets and the use of protein snacks. I added macrobiotic suggestions and training including the concept of complex and simple carbohydrates, the avoidance of animal food but when approaching the concepts of yin and yang I lost her Lord knows I wished for a macrobiotic center or even some macrobiotic counselors in town for indigent patients such as this to complete the dietary training. Despite what I would call decidedly incomplete dietary and macrobiotic training the patient improved She began to lose weight and inches. Now when Judy goes off the hypoglycemic diet (such as it is) she can recognize mood changes —she feels sluggish and has a dragged out feeling. Her medications have steadily been reduced as her functioning improves. She now has motivation to do new things and has made plans to return to school.

The second case, Alberta, is a middle-aged woman diagnosed as having manic depressive illness. She came to my department labeled as chronically mentally ill. She was expected to be on medication the rest of her life. Early in my treatment of her she complained that her family was angry since she was unable to lose weight. She had discussed this with her surgeon who had threatened to put her on diet pills since she seemed to have had no willpower of her own. We had succeeded in weaning her of most of her medication but at this time she feared she was losing her mind and felt she needed more medication. She reported to me that she experienced panic attacks and would feel driven to eat a candy bar. She questioned if she would not control her own mind and did this mean she would have another nervous break down.

I took a careful dietary history and then ordered a glucose tolerance test. She was not losing her mind, she was hypoglycemic During the test, at the exact time her blood sugar fell to its lowest level, she experienced one of her typical panic attacks and went to the hospital gift shop in search of a candy bar. To be sure, she was relieved to learn she was not going insane and that she could be treated by diet. Now when she slips off her hypoglycemic (quasi macrobiotic) diet, within an hour she notices she feels odd and numb. Then a half hour later she experiences a panic and an angry fit—once she threw things and broke a window. She does not do that now, she is convinced she can control her "mental illness" with diet and she does. Luckily I did not just pump her full of tranquilizers and leave her to flounder through life as she had.

These patients are but two of many hundreds of cases I am now learning could be successfully helped with appropriate diet, especially if it were macrobiotic. When I look into our busy waiting room and see patients drinking down another quart of cola I know they are using the drink as a current extreme trying to balance other extremes, at least for a moment.

As I began to work with a macrobiotic minds' eye with my patients, I began to search the medical literature for articles about macrobiotics. I was shocked to find so much negative information about the subject. In one computer literature search using MED-LINE, the National Library of Medicine's database, I found twenty-three articles about the macrobiotic diet, twenty-one of which were negative. These included articles like "Unproven Methods of Cancer Management—Macrobiotic Diets"[6] which stated: "After careful study of the literature and other information available to it, the American Cancer Society has found no evidence that treatment with macrobiotic diets results in objective benefit in the treatment of cancer in human beings. Lacking such evidence, the American Cancer Society would strongly urge individuals afflicted with cancer not to participate in treatment with macrobiotic diets. In addition, the more restrictive macrobiotic diets pose a serious hazard to health."

A second typically negative article appeared in *Oncology Nursing Forum* entitled "The Macrobiotic Diet: A Question of Nutrition."[7] The article states: "This Macrobiotic diet has been found to produce multiple nutritional deficiencies. Nutritional hazards documented in healthy people become even more apparent in those with disease. This article will state how the macrobiotic diet may compromise the nutritional status of the cancer patient and suggest strategies in counseling such patients." I was dismayed to find that the article went on to say: "Once a macrobiotic dietary pattern is identified, it is the nurse's responsibility to inform the patient of its associated hazards."

Where did this attitude come from I wondered. My answer

came from another widely quoted paper which appeared in the *Journal of the American Medical Association*[8] which was presented as a position statement of the Association's Council on Foods and Nutrition. The paper states: "The concepts proposed in *Zen Macrobiotics* constitute a major public health problem and are dangerous to its adherents. The dietary regimens proposed basically comprises ten diets, ranging from the lowest level (diet-3), which includes 10 percent cereals, 30 percent vegetables, 10 percent soup, 30 percent animal products, 15 percent salads and fruits, and 5 percent desserts, to the highest level (diet 7), which is made up of 100 percent cereals."

Having studied this I found myself saying, "Hey! This doesn't sound like the macrobiotic diet I know!" *The Macrobiotic Way* by Michio Kushi[9] states the *standard macrobiotic diet* consists of "50 to 60 percent whole grains and grain products; 20 to 30 per cent locally grown (when possible, organically grown) vegetables 5 to 10 percent beans and sea vegetables; 5 to 10 percent soups and 5 percent condiments and supplementary foods, including beverages, fish and desserts." As I pursued the rest of the negative medical articles I realized they referred usually to the *Zen Macrobiotic diet* and have inferred guilt by name association to any and all macrobiotic diets.

The good news comes from, of all places, the United States Congress. In a publication of the House of Representatives Subcommittee on Health and Long-term Care[10] it states: "the current macrobiotic diet . . . appears to be nutritionally adequate if the mix of foods proposed in the dietary recommendations are followed carefully. There is no apparent evidence of any nutritional deficiencies among current macrobiotic practices. The diet is consistent with the recently released dietary guidelines of the National Academy of Sciences and the American Cancer Society in regard to possible reduction of cancer risks."

The other positive article found in the literature review was an interesting little piece in the *British Journal of Clinical Psychology*[1] by Vicky Rippue entitled "Dietary Treatment of Chronic Obsessional Ruminations." Here the author reports: "Biochemical and clinical evidence supports the hypothesis that hypoglycemia secondary to inappropriate diet was the cause of the disorder

Dietary contributions to obsessional ruminations should probably be sought early in the assessment of such patients." Even though the diet used with this patient looked more like the quasi-macrobiotic diet my two patients were using, I found great pleasure in finding positive reference to mental illness, hypoglycemia, and dietary treatment.

Despite the controversy, at least in the conservative medical literature, I know the macrobiotic diet has much to contribute to the health and well-being of mental patients and people with all sorts of chronic diseases. As Michio Kushi and Edward Esko have stated in the book *Crime and Diet—The Macrobiotic Approach*[12],: "The standard macrobiotic way of eating is not designed for any particular person nor for any particular condition. It is designed for the purpose of maintaining physical and psychological health, and for the well-being of society in general. It further serves in many instances to prevent degenerative diseases and promote possible recovery."

This statement should go far to quiet the negative attack on macrobiotics from the medical community which seems to fear that macrobiotics claims it is a cure all and end all. Just as other health promoting and spiritually enhancing approaches have endured, macrobiotics has grown and matured to gain a clear and positive image today. My family now enjoys improved health and harmony as we continue to live the macrobiotic way. Somehow we must find a way to provide macrobiotic support to mentally ill persons. We need to perform scientific research and present clear and convincing evidence that macrobiotics can reduce the morbidity of mental illness and reduce the need for psychotrophic medication for the chronically mentally ill. One possible way to do this could be to set up and staff group homes for the mentally ill with macrobiotic staff (cooks and counselors) which are associated with psychiatric care providers who are sensitive to the patients' dietary needs and who will document data on the condition of these patients as they change their diets and lives.

As a final thought, I am reminded of the reaction of my 90-year-old grandmother in her nursing home when we went to eat lunch with her. All we could accept was the salad with no dressing and the vegetables with no butter. At that moment I pictured myself sitting there some fifty years from now trying to survive the food. We had better start planning for macrobiotic nursing homes and retirement communities now. Maybe they will be in place by the time we need them.

References

[1] Olinger, David. "Dispensing Drugs: A Delicate Problem," *Concord Monitor*, Concord, NH, Feb. 27, 1981

[2] *The American Heart Association Cookbook*, New York: David McKay Company, Inc., 1979.

[3] Wentworth, Josie A. *The Migraine Prevention Cookbook*, New York: Doubleday and Company, Inc., 1983.

[4] Spiegel, Hebert and Spiegel, David. *Trance and Treatment Clinical Uses of Hypnosis*, New York: Basic Books, Inc., 1978.

[5] Bell, Iris R. *Clinical Ecology*, Bolinas, California: Common Knowledge Press, 1982.

[6] Editors. "Unproven Methods of Cancer Management—Macrobiotic Diets," *CA* 34 (1): 60–63, Jan/Feb, 1984.

[7] Arnold, Cathy. "The Macrobiotic Diet: A Question of Nutrition," *Oncology Nursing Forum* 11 (3): May/June, 1984.

[8] Council on Foods and Nutrition. "Zen Macrobiotic Diets," *Journal of the American Medical Association* 218 (3): Oct. 18, 1971.

[9] Kushi, Michio. *The Macrobiotic Way*, Wayne, New Jersey: Avery Publishing Group, Inc., 1985.

[10] House of Representatives, Subcommittee on Health and Long-Term Care. "Quackery: a $10 Billion Scandal" Washington, DC: US Gov. Print Off, 1984: 66–8, 107; Committee Publication No. 98–435.

[11] Rippue, Vicky. "Dietary Treatment of Chronic Obsessional Ruminations," *British Journal of Clinical Psychology*, 22: 314–316, 1983.

[12] Kushi, M. et al. *Crime and Diet—The Macrobiotic Approach*, Tokyo/New York: Japan Publications, Inc., 1987.

Awakening to Common Sense

Guillermo Asis, M.D.

I was born in Argentina in 1948, and brought up with a diet particularly rich in beef and sugar, and poor in vegetables. As a matter of fact, my mother often tells me that as an infant I was given the juice from beef. This is nothing out of the ordinary in a culture in which the question how many times a day a person eats meat is more valid than how many times a week.

I completed medical school in 1975 when I decided to immigrate to this country. I studied immunology and virology at Georgetown University in Washington D.C. in 1976 until July 1977, and then started a four-year training program in internal medicine and cardiology at Tulane University in New Orleans.

Most people are unaware of the transformation that goes on in the individual over the period of being a medical student, intern, then resident. For the most part, the medical student is characterized by his/her good manners with patients. Once the process of post-graduate training starts, one's survival comes into question—a very demanding schedule often takes its toll on the respect and good manners which should be shown to patients. The former medical student has become a lot more impersonal, losing some of his humanity. In addition to this personal process, mistakes are bound to happen in a hospital. If one keeps an awake and critical perspective during medical training he or she will begin to question the system.

During medical training you are either confronted with situations of frustration such as the inability to help people with serious diseases such as cancer or AIDS, or with some occasional disaster which would never had occurred if the patient had been at home instead of admitted unnecessarily to the hospital and exposed to serious infections and/or expensive and often dangerous diagnostic procedures.

I was in this process of internal questioning, when in the spring of 1980, my best friend at the time, a doctor in his late twenties and in the same training program, was diagnosed as having cancer of the pancreas which spread to his liver. At first I was in disbelief. This was a disease that was supposed to be present only (or mostly) in persons aged fifty or older. Why my friend? He was much too young. And a doctor—this was not supposed to happen to us doctors. My friend was told that conventional medicine had nothing to offer him, that he would have a rather simple surgical procedure to avoid becoming jaundiced (turning yellow) and that he would be sent home.

Just by coincidence, during a rare evening at home, I watched a television program called *PM Magazine* in which Professor Jean Kohler described how he recovered from pancreatic cancer with the aid of macrobiotics.

My interest exploded at a moment that would change my life. Since a family member was a local producer for *PM Magazine*, I decided to go to the station and see the program again (and again). I called the Kohler's home, probably to check to see if he was a real person. Mrs. Mary Alice Kohler answered. Although she had words of encouragement, she said they could make no promise that it would work for my friend.

I would not believe this was a hopeless situation and spoke to my friend about macrobiotics. Unfortunately, in the midst of his despair, he did not see the opportunity and declined to follow the diet. His refusal was difficult for me to accept and I realized that it was probably due to a combination of factors. On the one hand, we had to acknowledge that in the culture in which we live, to have a diagnosis of cancer (and/or now, AIDS) is the closest thing to a death sentence.

And, outside of our personal beliefs, we are all ultimately part of the same culture and at some point or another, we shared the same beliefs. We grew up with them! In addition, being a doctor did not help my friend, rather, it was probably a detriment. After all, we, as doctors, know disease—or, think we do. We are taught that diet would not heal disease, and outside of perhaps diabetes or ulcers, diet would rarely be part of a doctor's advice at all.

I had to finally come to grips with the reality that it was his choice, independent of my good intentions. Looking back to those days, I think how surprising it was that he did not look for other alternatives, even if macrobiotics did not interest him. It is fair to say, however, that the general public's knowledge of alternative healing methods is very poor. Is it the government's responsibility to educate us? It would be a valuable service if organizations such as the American Cancer Society were to publish fair and non-judgmental descriptions of these methods.

By this time, I had gotten hold of a flyer which was sent to *PM Magazine* with an invitation to an upcoming Macrobiotic Program at Amherst College in Massachusetts. I did not think long (I was interested by then) and quickly booked a flight. I still do not know how I got the time off!

I spent a beautiful and peaceful late-August week at the Amherst Summer Program and got a sense of the possibility that macrobiotics offered. There were a variety of people there: students, teachers, and "friends of macrobiotics." I also had the opportunity to meet the Kohlers at the camp. They were a real inspiration.

Interestingly enough, however, despite the fact that the course was about healing, it was very noticeable that few doctors were present. I was very aware of the people at the camp who were seeking better health. There was something very different about these people that was not present in patients with similar conditions who I had just seen the previous week at the hospital. These people were vital, active, and had a certain happiness, despite their conditions. And they were full of hope. To this day, and regardless of how skeptical someone would be of macrobiotics, I see great value in following a healing method which infuses hope in a patient who would otherwise be in despair.

Another thing that I found striking was the food at the camp. There was something very peaceful and harmonious about the food served. The colorful presentation was a feast for the eyes. People as a rule do not make such a big deal about eating. Is it that we take for granted our process of nourishing and replenishing ourselves? Somehow there seems to be a gap between how much effort we put into nourishing ourselves and how much concern we seem to have for the end result: our health.

Soon after I returned to New Orleans I made the decision to move to Boston as soon as I completed my year of cardiology (in July of 1981). I intended to continue my macrobiotic education.

Needless to say, my thinking of disease and healing changed

substantially, and would go through a lot more changes in the years to come. I went from conversations with my father, while a medical student in Argentina, about how people practicing alternative healing methods were a bunch of quacks, to the time of my training in New Orleans when I often wondered how much good or harm we were really doing to our patients. Getting myself involved with macrobiotics came as a much needed ray of light with an open field of opportunities. It did not take long for me to have the chance to personally put my recently acquired knowledge to work. Two months after I returned from Amherst, I developed a kidney-stone attack. I had all the symptoms described in a medical textbook, all of them! The pain was unbearable. While colleagues were ready to administer heavy pain medications and admit me to the hospital for x-rays, I insisted upon only having applications of hot-compress preparations made from the juice of ginger root. I strongly suspect that some doctors thought I was crazy. As it turned out, I felt better than before the attack, with only three applications of the ginger compress during a 48-hour period. And I never had the problem again. I felt truly proud of not having taken even an aspirin or Tylenol during that episode.

Once in Boston I took two levels at the Kushi Institute's program which will always remain with me as an unforgetable learning experience. My diet, from the basic rudiments, mistakes, and guessing of the beginner underwent a transformation. Not only was the pace, the level of stress and competitiveness significantly different from medical school, at the Institute I had the sense of being vital at the end of the day, rather than feeling totally rundown, as I did with classes at medical school.

We learned many things at the Kushi Institute. From the basics of yin and yang, the theory of the five transformations, "new" ways of traditional diagnosis, a different approach to healing with food preparations, and shiatsu massage and external healing applications. Overall, the most important thing I learned was to get away from the stubborn and arrogant attitude learned in medical school and training, that only doctors know about healing. I also came to terms with how much we really do not know in the matter. It was crucial to redevelop common sense in diagnosing and making medical recommendations.

At this point, I was ready to participate in the healing of other people. I opened a holistic medical practice in Brookline with an acupuncturist and a chiropractor. Over the past seven years I have seen many patients from a new perspective of healing and hope. From this new angle, I have also seen how chronic degenerative diseases, like coronary disease and cancer, are dealt with by the medical community; which for the most part shows a total unawareness and disrespect for the effects of polluted and artificial dietary habits and regular exercise, as well as general attitude and life/relationships in connection with the origin and treatment of disease.

It seems to me, like a naturally unfolding story (I guess this is what conventional medicine calls the natural history of disease) to see how these medical conditions start from a childhood of baby formula and sugar, through years of drugs, to an adulthood of excesses in which the surfacing of heart disease and cancer should, far from showing up as a real surprise, be the expected end result of many years of poor judgment.

It is sad to see how stuck we are in our bad habits. Very often we seek a holistic approach for a chronic disease, like cancer or AIDS, when the disease is very advanced, while it would have been ideal to prevent it through macrobiotics and healthy living patterns. In the case of chronic heart disease, and coronary problems in particular, rather than seek alternative healing such as diet and exercise, most people affected are attracted to the efficiency and generally low risk of coronary artery bypass surgery.

We seem to have lost the common sense perspective of the fact that getting "new pipes" for blood to flow through is far from attacking the root of the problem, regardless of how much time it buys us. Not to mention that the infrequent, though possible, short- and long-term complications of this very involved surgical procedure may spoil the "fun" of beating the laws of nature; and of seemingly getting away with an eight-day hospital stay, a chest scar, and a large medical bill in exchange for years of excesses and abuse to one's body.

My personal experience with the use of macrobiotics (as well as acupuncture and homeopathy) has been the following: while on one hand it is the person/patient and his general attitude of life (which includes, though goes much beyond positive thinking) that remains the primary asset to ensure successful recovery of any illness, the use of the macrobiotic diet has made, in my experience, a major contribution in all of the cases I have seen of recovery from chronic disease.

It would be in many instances a process of re-education, learning to co-exist better with our environment and eating with the seasons, like our forefathers did, that will assist us in keeping healthy or regaining our health. I am always amazed to see how many people drink ice cold water or other liquid in the middle of winter and at the same time complain of having cold hands and feet. If we stop to think about it, it is a clear indication of how much we have lost common sense. A list of other obvious examples could go on for pages and pages. One such example is the situation with most supermarket food. In order to make it attractive and have a long shelf life, total disregard is given to the amount of colorants and preservatives used. Since it would take ten or more years to discover the implications these additives have in cancer or chronic diseases, why worry about it now?

We come now to the point that in the medical practice of the community at large, many issues come into question: 1) How free are people to personally choose the kind of treatment they want, particularly if the modality of approach and treatment departs from standard medical practice. Is the current level of freedom in this matter compatible with the free society that we advocate? 2) Why not have these options available within the medical insurance system since it is the patient who has been paying for the insurance anyway?

These considerations intertwine with deeper issues such as how do chronic degenerative diseases really relate to our daily eating habits? Yes, it is true that our thinking is changing in this area, but for the most part, these changes are happening at a very slow pace. This pace may be dictated in part by a very powerful food industry that is reluctant to change or let go of its share of the market.

Even deeper are the issues related to disease and cure: Does a cure really exist? Or, how do we know that we all do not have microscopic cancers that go into remission every day? This concept would define "cure" as a point of balance from which we come and go on a daily basis, and take away the heavy stigma that natural recovery is just a rarity or an impossibility.

Overall I am of the opinion that it pays off better to stay with this constant inquiry than to live in the fantasy of magic answers and magic cures. In this day and age, it is not common to find doctors, who when faced with a patient's questions, will have the courage to say plainly: "I don't know." Within the context of our cultural conditioning, far from accepting their honesty, or even that medicine as knowledge has limits, we will probably think the doctor does not know what he is doing, and therefore, we will change doctors.

We are presently going through a medical revolution which started just like any other revolution: from the bottom up. It will take more and more people exploring alternative healing, daily diet through macrobiotics, and demanding from their medical insurance companies, as well as from their government, preventive medicine, pollution control, and natural foods widely available across the country.

And, there is nothing special about such people. They do not have to be highly involved in politics, just common people who are tired of having attractive presentations of massively produced junk food at the cost of having their relatives and friends becoming increasingly afflicted with chronic degenerative illnesses. It could be said that they finally put two and two together. It is this kind of input from the general public that will force the scientific model to co-exist with the more experiential model that macrobiotics represents. This would be the road to "One Peaceful World" as Michio Kushi puts it.

To finish with some words of advice, I recommend that you truly take responsibility for your health and healing. If you stop to think about it, you really have little choice. This starts from caring for this wonderful gift given to us—our bodies— which are designed to survive and heal themselves, while surviving much abuse. Furthermore, when you go to a doctor for medical care, it may be in your own interest to have a realistic set of expectations. First of all you should realize that healing is really up to you, not to your doctor. The old way of speaking: "the doctor put me on this medication, or took me off that medication" is saying how little control we have in the general strategy of our own healing. Once you start seeing the doctor for what he or she is—a qualified advisor—you can make him or her your partner in a healthy, healing relationship. You will then create a new context for the practice of medicine.

So, how do you choose a medical practitioner who truly supports your unique healing process? Ask friends or organizations which you trust. Interview prospective doctors. Get a sense of how much they share your beliefs, or at least how much they are willing to respect your beliefs. And, once you have chosen him or her, come into the relationship with a new attitude. As the Bible and other great books teach us, the sky is the limit! Within the content of this new healing partnership with your doctor, you should be entitled to expect miracles.

It will take a major shift in our thinking, in the way doctors and hospitals communicate with us, and in the way we listen to them and interpret their message, to produce a transformation in the way we relate to disease. If we get really good at it, we may be able to eliminate disease all together. Just imagine a planet without the all-time burdens of world hunger, war and disease. As an important beginning, I recommend that you include your daily diet as a major part of this new thinking, explore *Macrobiotics* and learn about *Yin* and *Yang*. Its value has been well proven in the Orient over many centuries. As you are getting ready to start this new era you may want to keep in mind these words of Goethe:

"Whatever you can do, or dream you can, Begin it. Boldness has genius, power and magic in it."

PMS Is Not PMS

Helen V. Farrell, M.D.

Katharina Dalton, a British physician who first identified and studied the *Premenstrual Syndrome* (PMS), defines it as "the recurrence of symptoms in the premenstruum with absence of symptoms in the postmenstruum," and she says the diagnosis depends upon the timing of the symptoms and not on the symptoms themselves.

The Premenstrual Syndrome is the cluster of symptoms that occurs from one to fourteen days before the onset of menses. The symptoms can be both physical and psychological.

While the symptoms may vary from month to month as a woman reacts to the stresses of her personal life, family and work environments, they generally remain the same over a number of cycles. There is usually dramatic relief from the symptoms with the onset of the menstrual flow or at least within the first few days.

Katharina Dalton said that, in order for the symptoms to be classified as *PMS*, they had to disappear with the onset of the flow and that this timing was crucial to the diagnosis. However, I am not concerned when the symptoms come and go or how they are classified. If a woman has symptoms at any time, something is wrong.

The common symptoms that occur premenstrually are mood swings, irritability, depression, weepiness, anxiety, anger, a lack of concentration, judgment, and self-worth, decreased libido, fatigue, bloating, breast tenderness, headaches, acne, insomnia, food cravings, and dizziness. The list is endless. Furthermore, any other disease or condition can be aggravated at this time.

Other common complaints are sinus problems, flu-like symptoms, sore throat, itchy ears, constipation alternating with diarrhea, cold sores, vaginal discharge, and frequent urination.

In my practice I have found that women of all ages can have these problems from puberty until well after the menopause. It is more common, however, in the woman in her thirties. This is probably because the stresses of life have started to build up. Poor nutrition, lack of exercise, drugs, contraceptive pills, smoking, surgery, pregnancies, and breast-feeding have all added to the body's increasing inability to maintain biochemical balance while consuming a North American diet.

Usually, doctors tell women these symptoms are "just nerves" or "it's all in your head," or "you are a woman, grin and bear it." A lot of doctors routinely prescribe antidepressants or tranquilizers, assuming that the problem is most likely due to a Valium deficiency!

When I lecture on PMS, I usually begin by describing what I consider to be a normal menstrual cycle, since many women are unaware of what is normal and what is not. And, historically speaking, women seem to have accepted the fact that they must grin and bear the monthly pain and discomfort.

The length of the cycle should be regular, plus or minus two to three days, and roughly 25 to 35 days in length. On day one, the onset of menstruation, there should be no discomfort or cramps. The flow should start immediately, a continuous red flow with no clots. The flow should subside completely within three to five days. At ovulation there may be a mucus discharge, and a few twinges in the right or left lower abdominal area. The moods should not be out of control. About five to seven days before the period, there may be slight water retention and a decrease in energy. Women may need to be "spoiled" a little at this time as well.

I first started my PMS practice at the urging of a psychiatric colleague who noticed that a lot of the mood disorders experienced by the women she was treating were exacerbated by the premenstrual and menstrual phase. There was not much information on PMS available then, except for a few books by Katharina Dalton. She was convinced that the symptoms of PMS were brought on by an imbalance of estrogen and progesterone and found that progesterone suppositories were helpful in alleviating some of the symptoms. Other treatment included a few vitamins and restricting certain foods and beverages.

I was rather apprehensive those first few months dealing with this problem with such sketchy information, but over time, I tarted asking myself what this "disorder" was all about. Once I understood in more detail what a normal menstrual cycle should be like, (mainly by observation and personal experience), I came to the conclusion that PMS was really just an exaggeration of the normal physiological changes associated with menstruation. That is, certain biochemical imbalances in the body seemed to cause all the changes associated with menstruation to be blown out of proportion. Of course, if the patient had other problems or diseases, these conditions were also exaggerated premenstrually.

Why was it that the symptoms started at ovulation? I presumed that the hormone surge at this time was some sort of internal stress and that if the body was already compromised somehow then this added hormonal stress pushed the body "over the edge." This seemed sensible, because most patients experience dramatic relief of their symptoms once the period begins or once the hormones "shut off." So Dalton's concept of a hormonal basis for PMS seemed plausible. However, I discovered over time that the blood tests of PMS patients did not reveal any hormonal abnormality except in a small percentage (5 to 10%).

So I began to think that maybe it is the way the hormones are metabolized and regulated at the cellular level that is the crucial process. Therefore, if there is an imbalance of nutrients at the cellular level at any time, the hormones can hardly be expected to do their job properly. After all, the body is a biochemical "machine" and everything that is put into it by way of food, drink, and drugs is going to alter its biochemistry. The human species did not evolve over millions of years to go through the unpleasant symptoms it does every month. No other animal on earth experiences PMS.

Numerous theories have been put forward subsequently, attempting to explain the etiology of this disorder. Some of these are estrogen excess coupled with a relative deficiency of progesterone, altered carbohydrate tolerance and insulin secretion, vitamin deficiencies, prostaglandin imbalance, disruption of the renin-angiotension-aldosterone complex, impaired catecholamine metabolism, hypoglycemia, hormone allergy, fluid retention, and emotional illness.

I was quite excited when I first read the book *The PMS Solu-*

tion by Dr. Ann Nazzaro, as I thought it presented the problem clearly and logically. The book describes the current research into fatty acid metabolism and the clinical findings indicating that the delta-6-desaturase enzyme, which converts linoleic acid to gamma-linolenic acid, may be faulty in PMS sufferers.

Nazzaro sets out a nutritional program incorporating fatty acid supplements (evening primrose oil), vitamins, minerals, and some dietary advice. She notes good response in her PMS patients. It is understandable that fatty acid and vitamin supplements are helpful to a lot of women with premenstrual problems since stress, poor diet, and vitamin deficiencies will certainly interfere with the metabolism of fatty acids. In fact, these can contribute to the faulty metabolism of all other essential nutrients as well.

Before adopting Dr. Nazzaro's approach to therapy, I had been using vitamins and minerals and stressing some diet restrictions as my therapy for PMS. I found that moderate doses of vitamin B complex were helpful in increasing energy, improving mental outlook and decreasing bloating in some women. Also calcium and magnesium helped relieve menstrual cramps, while the addition of vitamins A and E and zinc regulated the menstrual flow and cycle length in some of my younger patients. Adding primrose oil to this regime certainly seemed to enhance the effectiveness of the vitamins and minerals. *However, I noted that over a three- to six-month period the effect of the supplements seemed to wear off.* Also, patients began complaining about the number of tablets they had to swallow, and the cost of such a regime.

I then decided to concentrate more on the nutritional causes of PMS.

I must add here that I do see male patients who have similar problems. Men's biological rhythms are probably controlled by hormones too, but in a much less obvious way. Nevertheless, the stress of modern living affects men equally, and perhaps at times, more severely than women.

Why do women develop PMS symptoms? I point out to my patients that the menstrual cycle is usually the first system in the body to change if an illness, stress or nutritional fault occurs. It

ands to reason that because, biologically, we exist to carry on
ie race, the reproductive system is extremely important to us.
herefore, a woman's body changes daily for this purpose. And a
iange in our menstrual cycle, no matter how small, reflects a
iange in a woman's biochemistry.

So, to return to my question, why do women develop
mptoms? Well, we are all familiar with the saying, "we are
hat we eat." This answers my question. It is very discouraging
iat the majority of the medical profession refuses to acknowledge
ie importance of the nutritional approach to the prevention and
:covery from disease.

We all know that the incidence of heart disease, cancer, arthritis,
iabetes, allergies, and mental disorders are on the rise in our
ociety despite the efforts of modern medicine. These diseases
e prevalent mainly in North America and Western Europe.
Iost of the rest of the world does not experience these disorders
i such large numbers because their diets are different. It is interest-
ig to note that the incidence of "North American" diseases is on
ie rise in some countries where the diet is becoming more
Westernized."

What happens at the cellular level then, determines how we
el mentally and physically. And the balance of nutrients we put
to our bodies determines what happens at the cellular level. I
ime to the conclusion that PMS is therefore a manifestation,
st, or our poor eating habits and second, of all the other stresses
modern day living.

In my practice, I initially try to determine the patient's stress
ad. I then emphasize the importance of exercise not only as
irt of the PMS therapy, but also as a consistent part of their
iily life. Exercise can help promote a sense of well-being and
ovide an outlet for excess energy. In addition to the well esta-
ished benefits of exercise, including improved uterine function,
e physiological benefits are extremely helpful in the premen-
rual phase when women are prone to feeling negative about
eir bodies.

I would now like to turn to some of the symptoms I see in my
actice and comment on my observations.

Katharina Dalton stressed the timing of the symptoms of PMS.

While symptoms can generally occur at any point in the cycle there are three patterns of timing that are most common.

A lot of women experience symptoms at ovulation for one to three days. They then disappear, only to recur with greater intensity five to seven days before menses. Some women only have symptoms for three to seven days premenstrually while others suffer from the time of ovulation until the menstrual flow begins about fourteen days. In most cases, there is dramatic relief from the symptoms within 24 to 48 hours of the onset of the flow.

One of the most common complaints women have is premenstrual mood swings. Most women tell me that they can cope with the numerous physical discomforts, but it is the psychological symptoms that upset them and their families the most. At ovulation many women feel as though a switch has suddenly been turned on and they can no longer control their emotions. They become weepy, irritable, angry, irrational, uncoordinated, tired, short-fused, and possibly even suicidal.

It is obvious that the hormonal influence is a big factor in the severity of these symptoms. Estrogen and progesterone are known to alter the glucose-insulin metabolism thereby causing potential hypoglycemia. If the diet contains food or beverages that lower the blood sugar, this adds further to the problem. The extreme fluctuation in blood sugar prevents the brain from getting the constant supply of glucose it needs and consequently the "animal brain" takes over. This can account for many of the above symptoms.

If we are under stress, (and women are under stress in the premenstrual phase) and consume sugar, then this causes changes in certain brain hormones which can produce nervous tension and fatigue. In addition, sugar and caffeine also trigger insulin release in excess of what the body needs, and the blood sugar subsequently drops.

A lot of patients think that sugar gives them the energy they need to get through the day. It does, in fact, steal their energy away. Michelle Harrison, in her book, *Self-Help for Premenstrual Syndrome*, sums it up well by saying that burning sugar for fuel is like using newspaper for heat—it burns easily with a bright flame then quickly dies out and you need more paper.

Therefore, by eliminating caffeine, sugar and other sweeteners, and eating small, frequent meals, the blood sugar can be stabilized. The mood swings are not as severe then. I have noted, however, that in some patients the mood swings do not disappear with dietary control. In these cases, I assume that external stresses, or perhaps underlying emotional problems are severe and consistent enough to trigger the premenstrual problems. It makes good sense, also, to schedule stressful events for other times in the cycle.

A woman may need about 500 calories a day more during the premenstrual phase. This means a general appetite increase. It does not mean specific food cravings. Because the North American diet is unbalanced and extreme, food cravings are common. Sugar cravings—and particularly chocolate cravings—are among the most common complaints in my practice. On a diet high in sugar, women will usually crave it more at a time when the blood glucose is low.

In macrobiotic theory, food cravings are explained by the overconsumption of extreme foods, that is, foods that are either too expansive or too contractive. If a contractive food is eaten, such as meat, cheese, or salt, the body will automatically crave expansive foods such as sugar to reestablish balance. As mentioned above, this phenomenon is enhanced premenstrually when the glucose metabolism is altered.

Bloating is a problem most women experience. A typical North American diet can cause constant bloating. I consider a small amount of bloating as normal premenstrual physiology. However, if bloating is excessive, it can lead to headaches, irritability, dizziness, hypersensitivity to light, lethargy, swollen extremities, and a general feeling of discomfort. Water retention is frequently caused by the overconsumption of salt. In addition, a diet high in refined carbohydrates triggers insulin release which prevents the kidneys from excreting salt. This also contributes to water retention. Therefore, when patients cut down their salt and sugar intake, their bloating is less.

Another bad habit patients have is consuming copious amounts of water. Of course, we constantly read about the health benefits of drinking a lot of water daily. But it stands to reason that if a person consumes six to eight glasses of water a day, plus tea, coffee and juices, and bloating is a problem, then perhaps the kidney cannot handle the load. The excess fluid is then deposited in the tissues. A lot of women urinate frequently and have to get up several times at night. This adds further stress at a time when it should be minimized.

Sore, swollen, lumpy breasts, beginning at ovulation and continuing until the menstrual flow, are a very common problem. In fact, in my practice, I estimate that 90 percent of my patients have tender breasts before their periods. For some patients this causes extreme discomfort. I used to use primrose oil and vitamin E for patients with this problem and noted a modest degree of success. However, it has become clear to me over the past few years that if women eliminate dairy products from their diet breast problems disappear within two to three months.

Annemarie Colbin, in her book *Food and Healing*, indicates that the consumption of dairy products appears to be strongly linked not only to breast discomfort, but also to other disorders of the female reproductive system such as ovarian tumors, cysts, vaginal discharge, infections, menstrual cramps, and heavy flow. She indicates that by eliminating foods that relate to the reproductive system of animals, such as milk and milk products, eggs, and the meat of animals raised on estrogens, the problems disappear.

Another frequent complaint is headaches. Premenstrual headaches are extremely common and seem to be associated with water retention, fatigue, and stress. I have found that the elimination of dairy foods from the diet has been one of the most important factors in alleviating migraine headaches. It is also essential to reduce water-retaining foods as well as those causing hypoglycemia.

A lot of patients wake up with headaches. This group seems to experience unusual drops in blood sugar during the night. By reducing caffeine, sugar, and other sweeteners and by eating complex carbohydrates, this problem can be alleviated.

Most people I see tend to be constipated and have a history of hemorrhoids or other bowel dysfunction. "If the bowels don't work properly, then nothing else will" has been one of my favorite expressions for some time. I usually explain to my patients that the bowels are like a central processing unit. Everything that goes into the body is processed there. If they do not operate properly, then the body cannot assimilate the nutrients it needs on a regular basis. A lot of people use laxatives or add fiber to their diet. Bran is the "in thing" these days. Why not eat the whole grain instead of just parts of it?

The other common cause of constipation is the overconsumption of dairy products. Once patients eliminate these from their diet, they have regular and more frequent bowel movements. It is the mucus from dairy products that interferes with bowel function causing constipation, diarrhea, gas, bloating, and hemorrhoids. Poor bowl function is also related to poor skin.

Most people do not understand the connections among the various systems of their body. They treat themselves, as does the majority of the medical profession, as a disconnected assortment of symptoms and problems.

I have always suspected that the skin directly reflects what goes on inside the body. I am amused at a dermatologist's approach to skin disorders. While they may notice a modest success in their treatments, they completely ignore the internal state of affairs.

Macrobiotics has certainly helped me understand the physiology associated with poor skin and the distribution of markings, pimples, and blemishes. I generally tell my patients that poor skin is a reflection of what goes on in the gastro-intestinal tract and is therefore directly related to what goes into the mouth. There is no doubt about the connection between sugar intake and pimples. But I have also recently discovered, through macrobiotic readings, that the elimination of animal protein, along with sugar, clears up the skin remarkably well. It is interesting to note that when patients start to alter their diets, their skin can become worse during the first few months. I presume this is the discharge phase or "healing crisis."

Most women note a few pimples around the mouth or chin area before a period. This is understandable, since, in Oriental diagnosis, this area represents the reproductive organs. Again, this illustrates how hormones can intensify biochemical imbalances.

Most people I see are unwilling to become vegetarians. Therefore, I deal with their skin problems by at least insisting they eliminate dairy products, red meat and sugar from their diets.

It is worthwhile mentioning the menopause here because, as with PMS, the symptoms associated with this time of life are merely a reflection of the poor nutritional status of a woman's body. Menopause is a natural event. If this is so, why do so many women suffer for years with numerous complaints? With the change in the ovaries, the decrease in hormone production, and the associated physiological changes, it is a great internal stress. It stands to reason, then, if the body is already operating in a compromised condition, any added stress is going to cause symptoms to appear. Therefore, the symptoms of menopause are like those of PMS, and this means that we deal with them in exactly the same way: with diet modification.

I see teenagers with the same problems that women have in their thirties and forties. It is sad that a lot of young girls suffer with severe menstrual cramps, vomiting, dizziness and headaches, and miss one to two days of school every month. In addition, they may have poor skin, fatigue, and mood swings. The effect of poor nutrition seems to manifest itself at puberty, a time when there is great internal change or stress.

I remember that as a child I had numerous coughs, colds, ear infections and often took antibiotics. In spite of losing my tonsils and my adenoids (twice, I may add), I was always sneezing and was very congested at night. The doctor said I was allergic to feathers. So I slept with a plastic bag on my pillow. This did not help. My skin was always bad. I was overweight, and when my periods started they were extremely painful. I also developed classical migraine headaches. I used nasal spray constantly for many years and always coughed in the morning. Chronic vaginal discharge and yeast infections were common.

Of course, this all fits in with my passion for milk and other dairy products. I could not believe the difference in my sinus problem after I stopped eating dairy food for only a very short time. It was miraculous.

My father has also suffered severely from nasal congestion, post nasal drip and the usual clearing-the-throat cough. He also had nasal polyps. Injections and drugs gave him some short-term relief. When I finally convinced him to stop dairy products, he could not believe the change. The first thing he said to me was, "I can smell again!"

I have suffered from classical migraine headaches since I was eleven years old, experiencing scintillating scotomas, dysphasia, transient parasthesias, and vomiting: the classic textbook case. Although I did not notice the pattern at the time, the headaches were probably cyclical in nature and more prevalent during my period. Extensive neurological testing failed to come up with anything and, of course, traditional drug therapy did not alleviate the incredible pain. As I got older, I noticed that the headaches were much less frequent but usually occurred after some severe stress. For the past five years, I have been headache free and account for this by my reduction of dairy food, regular exercise, and generally better lifestyle habits.

Then, last July I was talking to a patient and suddenly experienced flashing lights in my left visual field. I also felt rather dizzy. I knew this was a migraine aura. The visual impairment became progressively worse, so I cancelled my appointments and went home. On my way, I began to think about the mechanism of this headache. It is vascular dilatation, a very "expansive" type of headache, in macrobiotic terms. Therefore I decided I should consume something more "contractive."

By the time I got home twenty minutes later, I could barely see, and the pounding migraine pain was just starting. I headed straight for the pantry and the *umeboshi* plum paste. I had been reading about this condiment and its "contractiveness," so I thought I would experiment and see if it worked or not. After about two teaspoons and within two minutes, the visual symptoms disappeared dramatically.* I could not believe it! I decided to lie down for a while as I was feeling a little weak, but I was extremely hopeful that maybe I had managed to prevent this headache attack and many hours of suffering. A hint of a headache remained but it never fully developed. Every twenty minutes or so, I con-

---

* For an explanation of the uses of umeboshi plum, please see *Macrobiotic Home Remedies* by Michio Kushi, edited by Marc Van Cauwenberghe, M.D., Japan Publications, 1985.

sumed more plum paste. In the meantime I rested and relaxed. Within two hours I got up, feeling completely normal with no headache, nausea or tingling. I thought, "I am now going to believe everything I read about macrobiotic healing!"

In my experience with well over 1,000 patients in the past few years, I have come to realize that one of the most widely damaging foods in the North American diet is dairy products. I always tell my patients that milk is for babies and cow's milk is for baby cows! We do not look, think, grow, or behave like cows so why are we drinking their milk?

The introduction of cow's milk at an early age can certainly account for numerous problems. Babies that are colicky or develop diarrhea when introduced to cow's milk are giving us a big clue. Why do we fail to pay attention? As a child grows and consumes dairy products, he may develop numerous upper-respiratory problems such as tonsillitis, frequent colds, chronic nasal congestion, runny nose, ear infections or asthma. He may also have headaches, insomnia, or be hyperactive. Parents may assume he has some sort of allergy but they usually ignore the fact that it may be food related.

As the child grows older, he may develop skin problems such as eczema and if female, have extremely painful and erratic menstrual cycles. He or she may be tired, lethargic, overweight, or have dark shadows under the eyes. Again, the symptoms may change over time but the effect of the continued dairy intake will cause various problems throughout life.

The most common problems I see related to dairy products are sinus congestion, headaches, ear infections, dizziness, and post nasal drip and coughing, especially upon awakening. Breast tenderness, vaginal discharge, ovarian cysts, painful periods, and fatigue are the most common female complaints.

Many patients have been told they have what the medical profession labels *Irritable Bowel Syndrome*. Patients think this a disease. Doctors label it as such because they do not know what causes it. They give it a name and treat it with drugs. The elimination of dairy products from the diet relieves this problem.

It was a patient who first introduced me to macrobiotics. I had heard the term before but really did not know too much about it. She suggested some books, and since at this time I was personally interested in improving my eating habits, I was anxious to learn more. My first macrobiotic book was *Introducing Macrobiotic Cooking*, by Wendy Esko. Reading the introductory chapters was very enlightening. It all made so much sense to me. Having had medical training and the opportunity to see and talk to hundreds of patients about their bodies, I knew that I had to read more on this subject. Then I read Michio Kushi's books, *Natural Healing Through Macrobiotics* and *How to See Your Health*, and a whole new world of medicine opened up for me.

I not only began applying some of my new-found knowledge to my patients, but I also began to cook macrobiotic foods for myself. Although my diet had not been totally unhealthy up to this point, my eating habits were somewhat erratic and I did have sugar binges.

After one month of eating macrobiotic food and stopping my vitamins, I felt worse than I had for a long time. I got an extremely bad cold, and was physically and mentally run down. Of course, this was all part of the discharge and healing phase, but I had a difficult time understanding this concept then and the fact that the food-preparation time did not fit into my schedule sent me slowly back to my old eating habits.

Over the past year and a half, along with my continued reading, and applying macrobiotics to patient care, I have become convinced that this type of approach to nutrition was the one that not only I, but everyone else, should be following. However, it is very difficult to introduce the average North American to macrobiotic cooking. Certainly, helping them decrease their consumption of meat, dairy foods, sugar, caffeine, and refined salt is one big step forward.

After taking some cooking classes and attending a macrobiotic conference, I have become a lot more organized in my approach to this way of eating and lifestyle. I have been more effective also in helping patients make dietary adjustments based on my own experiences. I advise my patients to allow some "fun food" in their diet from time to time so they do not feel deprived and then feel guilty if they "cheat." The desire to "cheat" will decrease naturally over time anyway.

I have come a long way professionally and personally in my approach to PMS and other related problems. I used to believe that the only real cure for PMS was pregnancy. Naturally, the cyclical occurrence of symptoms disappears during pregnancy. However, there are about thirty to forty hormones secreted at that time that can often mask the fact that the body is biochemically out of balance to start with. The pregnancy will add greater stress to the body and most likely make symptoms worse later on when the periods return.

PMS is not PMS. It is not a disease or a syndrome. It is merely a collection or focus of symptoms that occur in the female body as a result of stress, especially nutritional stress.

Although some women have found vitamin therapy to be temporarily helpful, it is not a fundamental solution. The elimination or at least the decrease in the consumption of caffeine, refined salt, sugar, alcohol, dairy products, and meat helps everyone increase their vitality and decrease their symptoms regardless of what they may be, and can serve as a preliminary step toward more complete dietary change.

In our society today, many women find it difficult to make dietary adjustments, particularly when their families resist the change. If they can at least become more aware of how the food they eat affects their mind and body, then they will have taken a big step forward in achieving an optimal menstrual cycle and good health.

References

Colbin, A., *Food and Healing*. New York: Ballantine Books, 1986.

Dalton, K., *The Premenstrual Syndrome And Progesterone Therapy*. Second Edition. Chicago: Year Book Medical Publishers, 1977.

Harrison, M., *Self-Help for Premenstrual Syndrome*. New York: Random House, 1982.

Kushi, M. *How To See Your Health: Book of Oriental Diagnosis*. Japan Publications Inc., 1982.

Kushi, M., *Natural Healing Through Macrobiotics*. Japan Publications Inc., 1978.

Lauersen, N., *Premenstrual Syndrome and You*. New York: Simon and Schuster Inc., 1983.

Nazzaro, A., Lombard, D., Horrobin, D., *The PMS Solution*. Eden Press, 1985.

Macrobiotics, Nutrition and Disease Prevention

Terry Shintani, M.D., J.D., M.P.H.

Introduction

When I first arrived in Boston to study for a Masters in nutrition, I also decided to take some classes at the Kushi Institute (K. I.) on macrobiotics. In those classes at the K. I. we were all asked to introduce ourselves. After I introduced myself as a physician, one of my classmates turned to me with a puzzled look and asked, "don't you find this a little contrary to your profession?" I answered that I found that medicine and macrobiotics were actually consistent with each other in many ways.

I see macrobiotics and modern science as two ways of looking at the same truth. One from the large "macro" view, a more holistic but less precise view, and the other from a "micro" view, a more precise, analytical view but a somewhat narrower perspective. There are many aspects of macrobiotic philosophy that Western science finds controversial at this time. But even this controversy is consistent with macrobiotics because macrobiotics teaches that one should adopt a perspective of "non-credo"—that is, do not blindly believe what is said. And in spite of some areas of controversy, I think it is important to look at the positive aspects of a philosophy that teaches people responsibility for their own health and attempts to promote happiness, freedom, and peace.

Furthermore, from the research of medical literature that I have done, I find that there are a surprising number of teachings of macrobiotics that are substantiated by modern science. Like you, the reader, I am one who is seeking the truth—the truth about life and how best to heal myself and others. This is one reason I became a physician. It is also one reason I am interested in macrobiotics—to see where these two approaches come together.

In this short essay, I would like to share with you my perspective on macrobiotics and a few of the many areas where I find that modern science and macrobiotics are in fact consistent with each other.

Personal Experience with Macrobiotics

My interest in macrobiotics started approximately twelve years ago when one of my best friends who was teaching English in Japan learned about macrobiotics and shared this philosophy with me. There were many claims by people about what could be accomplished through macrobiotics that aroused my curiosity. What interested me most at that time was the claim that people who were on a macrobiotic diet could sleep four to five hours and feel rested. I was about to enter law school in those days and it was very important to me to be able to study into the night and still wake up fresh. To my surprise I was able to feel rested with five to six hours of sleep after eating macrobiotically for just a few weeks. I had previously been requiring eight to nine hours.

While I realize there is no proof that it was the diet that actually caused this decrease in sleep requirement, this nonetheless made me even more curious about macrobiotics. I later found that there is scientific evidence that a low fat, high complex carbohydrate diet can improve REM (Rapid Eye Movement) sleep which could explain this phenomenon.[1]

Another of the many reasons I started on a macrobiotic diet was for health reasons. I wanted to avoid cancer and heart disease later in life. This led me to another aspect of the philosophy that had a deeper impact on me. It was the macrobiotic approach to illness. In essence, the macrobiotic perspective takes into account the whole person in the full context of his or her environment when evaluating illness. I found that this perspective was similar to the teachings of a well-known ancient Western physician, Hippocrates who said:

Whoever wishes to investigate medicine properly should

proceed thus: in the first place to consider the seasons of the year . . . then the winds, the hot and the cold, . . . One should consider most attentively the waters which the inhabitants use, . . . and the mode in which the inhabitants live, and what are their pursuits, whether they are fond of drinking and eating to excess, and given to indolence, or are fond of exercise and labor.[2]

Macrobiotic philosophy takes the position that in order to maximize health, one should be in harmony with the environment—and that one's closest contact with the environment is with food. In fact, it was pointed out that the molecules of one's food actually become the molecules of the person eating it. Thus, in order to maintain this harmony, to avoid certain diseases and to be as healthy as possible, one of the most important things a person can do for his or her health is to select foods properly. I was so intrigued with this concept that I wanted to learn more about this from a scientific perspective.

To my surprise there were very few physicians concentrating on a nutritional approach to disease. I felt that this was an important area that needed more emphasis and it became one of the major reasons I decided to become a physician and a nutritionist. This perspective has stayed with me throughout my medical training.

Nutrition and Evolution

In general, the macrobiotic diet as I understand it today is a nutritionally adequate diet for most people (with a few areas of controversy which I discuss below). This has been studied and published in the *Journal of the American Dietetic Association* in 1975.[3] Contrary to the belief of many nutritionists, the macrobiotic diet is not represented by the "number seven" diet composed of only brown rice, miso soup, and *bancha* tea. The standard macrobiotic diet is instead rich in variety and is a diet that was practiced by all major civilized cultures through the history of

mankind. In fact, the traditional way of eating that mankind ha
followed throughout the ages is a repeated theme in the descrip
tion of the macrobiotic diet.

Looking at the dietary patterns throughout the evolution o
mankind to find the ideal diet for mankind is not just an Easter
"macrobiotic" perspective. It has also been the interest of man
prominent Western scientists. There is a great deal of logic in thi
approach. It makes sense that available food sources play an im
portant part in the evolution of living organisms. The reasonin
behind this notion is that those members of a species who ha
the body chemistry and structure to function best on the availabl
food supply, physically, mentally, socially, and in reproductio
were the members who survived and propagated. This idea ha
been supported even at the molecular level by the study of DN/
in various species.[4] In fact, Dr. Munro states that:

> A defensible case can be made for the view that the mai
> driving force in the evolution of animals from the most pri
> mitive forms onward has been the supply of nutrients in th
> environment.[5]

If one accepts this view that nutrition is indeed the main drivin
force in the evolution of human beings, then the conclusion tha
humans are adapted to and function best on the foods on whicl
they evolved is a natural one. Thus, the principle of looking to
evolution that is behind the macrobiotic diet is a scientifically
sound one. Since every major culture in the history of mankinc
had a diet that was principally whole grain, it seems quite reason
able that a whole-grain-based diet is indeed the "natural" diet o
mankind.

Some scholars do raise the question as to what era in the history
of mankind should we examine to find the "natural" diet o
human beings. A recent article published in the *New Englana
Journal of Medicine* entitled "Paleolithic Nutrition" suggests
that we should look to paleolithic man's diet as a guide. The
authors speculate that since man has existed as a unique species
for over a million years and since agriculture and grain-centered
diets may have developed no more than roughly ten thousand

years ago, we should look to the pre-agricultural diets as the "natural" diet of mankind. This would be the diet of the hunter-gatherer. Such a diet would be high in wild meats and wild vegetables and very low in grains. While the high-meat content may sound unhealthy, it is still much different from the standard American diet which contains about 40 percent. In fact experts believe that the paleolithic diet contained only about 20 percent fat owing to the low-fat content of wild animals. Wild animals are estimated to contain roughly 4 percent fat whereas domesticated animals that we eat today contain 30 percent to 40 percent fat. In addition, because wild animals feed in the wild, they contain much higher amounts of omega-three fatty acids which have been shown to have protective value against heart disease.

No one can really say what is truly the "natural" diet of mankind except to say that we have shown remarkable adaptability to surviving on foods available in almost any niche in the world. We can only speculate what mankind's ideal diet might be based on information available from history, science, anthropology and various other disciplines.

From a medical perspective, a grain-centered diet makes sense. A macrobiotic grain-centered diet is low in fat, high in complex carbohydrates, and high in fiber. All these aspects of a grain-centered diet will reduce the risk of many diseases including the two biggest killers of Americans, cardiovascular disease and cancer.

From an evolutionary perspective, following the grain diet of post-agricultural man makes sense because evolution not only takes time but also takes large numbers of the members of a species to provide genetic variety. When the total number of human beings that ever existed on earth is considered, the best estimates show that more than half the earth's human population has lived in post-agricultural times. This means that in terms of numbers, there has been more opportunity for genetic adaptation for humans in post-agricultural times when grains were the principal food than in paleolithic times when man was a hunter-gatherer. Moreover, truly modern human beings did not appear until approximately 30,000 years ago. This also suggest that we should look at the more recent diets of mankind as the ideal diet for modern man and perhaps the hunter-gatherer diet as the ideal diet for ancient man.

The debate could go on and on. However, as I stated earlier little can be said for certain regarding what the ideal diet for mankind is except that man has been able to adapt to food sources from almost any niche in the world. The interesting thing is that this idea is consistent with macrobiotics. One of the basic principles of macrobiotics is to eat foods in season and in the appropriate climate. That is, eating according to the niche in the world that he or she occupies. This makes maximum use of any genetic adaptability that may have developed over the millenia.

Nutritional Adequacy of Macrobiotics

As with any diet, anyone who is ill or on medication should seek the advice of a physician before embarking on a significant dietary change. However, for the majority of the population, a macrobiotic diet based on current recommendations when followed carefully supplies all the essential nutrients (with a few areas of controversy discussed below) necessary for good health. In fact, the current macrobiotic recommendations provide a diet that is very close in composition to that which has been set forth by the U. S. Senate Select Committee on Nutrition.[6] In addition, numerous studies indicate that it will help to prevent cardiovascular disease and certain kinds of cancer.

Calcium: One of the nutrients in controversy in the macrobiotic diet is calcium. The concern is raised largely because dairy food is not part of the macrobiotic diet, and dairy food is considered by many nutritionists as our best source of calcium. There is additional concern because of the high rates of osteoporosis in this country. According to some studies, the macrobiotic diet contains about 640 mg of calcium per day. This exceeds the World Health Organization's recommendations of 400 to 500 mg of calcium per day although it does not meet the current RDA of 800 mg or the proposed recommended levels of 1,000 to 1,500 mg. One should recognize that the RDA is not meant to be construed as a minimum requirement but rather a level that will safely cover practically all healthy people. In other words, there is some degree of speculation even among good Western scientists as to what an adequate calcium intake should be and a hefty safety factor is built into the RDA. Thus, whether the 640 mg of calcium in a macrobiotic diet should or should not be regarded as "deficient" is controversial at least from a worldwide perspective.

Many people believe that osteoporosis can be prevented by eating dairy food or by taking calcium supplements. At this point, there is conflicting data as to whether dairy food or calcium supplements will improve calcium balance and prevent osteoporosis. Studies are now underway to establish or discount this theory. However one should recognize that most countries have calcium intakes of 500 mg or less and many of these countries have less osteoporosis than the United States. In addition, most Asian and African countries have much lower dairy intakes than the United States and yet have lower rates of osteoporosis than we do.

Vitamin B12: Another area of controversy regarding the macrobiotic diet is its vitamin B_{12} content. Vitamin B_{12} is an essential nutrient which contributes to the formation of red blood cells. It is also important in the maintenance of *myelin*, which is the sheath around nerves which aids in the proper conduction of nerve impulses. Dietary B_{12} content is an issue because it is a substance not found in plants. Some scholars reason that this is an indication that man was not intended to be a strict vegetarian. Indeed no major culture on earth was purely vegetarian (although animal food was not a daily food for most cultures).

However, B_{12} is only required in minute quantities. The official USA daily recommendation is 3 micrograms or three millionths of a gram. It is estimated that the average person has three years worth stored in his or her body. Adequate amounts can be found in certain sea vegetables and fermented foods because B_{12} is produced by the microorganisms that are found in these foods. Sea vegetables and fermented foods are recommended daily in the macrobiotic diet. This makes macrobiotics superior to some pure vegetarian diets which do not have similar recommendations. In addition, the macrobiotic diet is not strictly vegetarian as occasional animal foods (preferably seafood) are generally permitted. This aspect makes the macrobiotic diet consistent with the anthropological perspective that no major culture was purely vegetarian. It also makes the macrobiotic diet consistent with the perspective than man's B_{12} requirement implies that humans were intended to eat animal food albeit a small amount.

Prevention of Disease

In the last ten or fifteen years, modern science in its own way has been increasing its emphasis on a larger view of the world by it increased reliance on epidemiological studies of chronic diseases One of the conclusions of such studies is that we are now under going an epidemic of heart disease, diabetes, and some cancers In fact, six of the ten leading causes of death in the United States are diet related. Recognizing these facts, the Senate Select Committe on Nutrition made an attempt to address this problem and set forth a set of dietary goals for the United States in 1977 and revised them in 1980. In this document, Dr. D. Mark Hegsted of the Harvard School of Public Health stated:

> The diet of the American people has become increasingly rich—rich in meat, other sources of saturated fat and chole sterol, and in sugar. . . . The risks associated with eating this diet are demonstrably large. The question to be asked, therefore is not why should we change our diet but why not? . . . Ischemic heart disease, cancer, diabetes and hypertension are the diseases that kill us. They are epidemic in our population. We canno afford to temporize. We have an obligation to inform the public of the current state of knowledge and to assist the public in making the correct food choices. To do less is to avoid our responsibility.[7]

In order to minimize the risk of these diseases this report re commends reducing fat, simple sugar, and cholesterol intake increasing the amount of complex-carbohydrate intake, and in creasing dietary-fiber intake. A macrobiotic diet is similarly low in fat, sugar and cholesterol, and high in complex carbohydrates and fiber. What I find fascinating is that both macrobiotics and modern science in pursuing an optimal diet for health arrived at similar conclusions from two entirely different approaches.

Cardiovascular Disease: The greatest killer of Americans today is cardiovascular disease including strokes, heart disease, and other problems related to poor circulation. Approximately 40 percent of all Americans die of cardiovascular disease. One of the best ways to minimize this is by reducing our intake of cholesterol and saturated fats. Studies indicate that there is a direct correlation between cholesterol and death from cardiovascular disease. Dr. William Castelli of the well-known Framingham Study has pointed out that a one percent change in cholesterol is associated with a two-percent change in risk of heart disease. In fact in the Framingham Study, no one with a cholesterol level below 150 died of a heart attack.

The standard macrobiotic diet is very low in cholesterol and fats. Thus, practically anyone on a macrobiotic diet will likely reduce his or her risk of cardiovascular disease. This was substantiated by a study done at Harvard University by Dr. Frank Sacks and his associates which was published in the *New England Journal of Medicine* in 1975.[8] In that study, the average cholesterol level in macrobiotic subjects was found to be 126 whereas the average level in controls from the Framingham Study who ate the standard American diet was 184.   This is not surprising as it had been shown in 1981 that a change from the standard American diet to a vegetarian diet produced a change of cholesterol level of 30 to 100 mg per dl within two weeks.[9]

Cancer: While there are many forms of cancer that are associated with certain macro- and micronutrients, probably the clearest correlation is between dietary fat and certain forms of cancer. Breast cancer is probably the most notable example of this. Epidemiological studies have shown that countries that have a low-fat diet have low incidences of breast cancer. In fact there is almost a linear correlation between the amount of dietary fat and the incidence of breast cancer among countires.[10]

One of the best studies on this issue done recently surveying nearly 90,000 women indicated that there is no correlation between breast cancer and dietary fat. However, in this study, the lowest category of fat intake among these women was 30 percent fat. This taken together with other epidemiological studies could be interpreted as suggesting that one needs to have a dietary fat intake lower than 30 percent to have a preventive effect on breast cancer. This interpretation is supported by the fact that the countries with the lowest breast-cancer rates in Caroll's article had fat intakes of as low as 15 percent. It is also supported by the fact that low-fat diets reduce four of the risk factors for breast cancer, namely obesity, serum cholesterol, estrogen, and prolactin.

As for other kinds of cancer, there is a fairly strong correlation between high dietary fat and low dietary fiber with cancer of the colon. The macrobiotic diet should help change these risk factors as well as it is low in fat (about 15 to 20 percent) and high in fiber.

Another example of how macrobiotics helps prevent cancer is found in the relationship of vitamin A in the form of beta carotene and certain forms of cancer. Recent studies have pointed to vitamin A or *beta carotene*, (the precursor of the active form of vitamin A, *retinol*) as being protective against certain cancers. In Norway, one study showed that men who had a higher than average consumption of vitamin A had less than half the rate of lung cancer as did those who consumed less vitamin A. Similarly, studies in Japan, Singapore, and the United States have shown an inverse relationship between vitamin-A intake in the form of beta carotene and lung cancer. Other studies have shown a similar relationship between vitamin-A intake and cancers of the bladder, stomach, and breast.

A macrobiotic diet is very high in vitamin A in the form of beta carotene. Thus, based on these studies a macrobiotic diet should help prevent lung cancer and other forms of cancer as well.

In the conclusion of this section of the article on this study, the author stated that "it is possible that constituents of green and yellow vegetables other than carotene actually reduce cancer incidence."[11] In other words, in order to be sure of the observed anti-cancer benefits of beta carotene, one would best eat the whole food just in case some other micronutrient in that food was causing the anticancer effect. Once again, this is a conclusion consistent with macrobiotic recommendations.

Obesity: There is fairly good evidence that a diet that is high in fiber and complex carbohydrates and low in fat will help someone lose weight and keep that weight off. These are characteristics of the macrobiotic diet and thus it is reasonable to assume that macrobiotics is good for weight loss. Studies have shown that fiber helps improve satiety or the feeling of satisfaction at a lower calorie level. In addition, dietary fiber helps to slow absorption of food so that the glycemic (blood sugar) curve would stay steady longer. This would tend to make a person satisfied longer and thus eat fewer calories in the long run.

Another factor that would make macrobiotics good for weight loss is in its low-fat content. Dietary fats are the highest in calories of any nutrient with about nine calories per gram. Brown rice is by comparison about 1.1 calories per gram. Just by calorie concentration alone it would be much easier to lose weight on a low-fat diet such as macrobiotics than on a high-fat diet. In experiments with mice which were allowed to eat as much as they wanted, the percentage of dietary fat determined how many of them became obese. Since a macrobiotic diet is low in fats, it should be conducive to weight loss based on these studies.

One should remember that obesity is a multi-factorial problem. Exercise and mental aspects need to be considered. Macrobiotics encourages a positive mental attitude and regular physical activity. And since the macrobiotic diet is low in energy density (low in calories per gram) because of the high-fiber and low-fat content, it is a reasonable conclusion that such a diet would be helpful in a weight-loss program. In studies done on low energy density diets, it has been shown that people feel more satisfied with fewer calories and maintain weight loss over time with such a diet.

There have been a large number of recoveries of "incurable" diseases, including cancer, associated with this diet. There have been numerous books about case histories of recovery from cancer. The recovery of Dr. Anthony Satillaro who recovered from metastatic prostatic cancer and Elaine Nussbaum who recovered from metastatic cancer of the uterus, and Jean Kohler who recovered from pancreatic cancer are some well-known examples. There are many other cases of recovery from cancer that are unpublished. This issue is much more controversial than the issue of the preventive value of a macrobiotic diet.

This is an area in which everyone can improve and learn from modern medicine. So often the evidence used for support of alternative approaches to healing is based on single cases or anecdotes. There is a maxim that I learned in medical school that pertains to this: "Beware the doctor who cites a single case." In other words, be very wary about what a physician says if it is based on a single case alone because there are many pitfalls to conclusions not based on an adequate number of cases. For example, a single case may be unique or the observer may have affected the outcome or may be biased in reporting the results. More studies need to be done to verify or change many of the claims made based on macrobiotic principles. The lack of such studies is one of the reasons that macrobiotics has not been well accepted by the medical community in the past. However, this too is changing. Studies are now being done on the relationship between macrobiotics and various diseases including cancer, one of them notably by Dr. Lawrence H. Kushi.

However, anecdotal examples and books are not without value. These serve as excellent guidelines for research such as those by Dr. L. H. Kushi and Dr. F. Sacks mentioned above. In addition, in cases where there is no effective treatment (i.e., where effective treatment is not avoided) as in most kinds of advanced cancer, I feel that an informed choice to pursue a safe, inexpensive approach based on documented histories is a reasonable course to pursue when conventional alternatives have been exhausted.

Moreover, there is now a growing body of scientific evidence that may support the value of diet in the palliation or recovery of some forms of cancer. For example, one recent study has suggested that women with advanced breast cancer who are on a low-fat diet may survive longer than those who are not on such a diet.[12] While this is not conclusive, confirmation of such results could have a major impact on the treatment of cancer in the future.

I think a word of caution about the use of diet in cancer is warranted. One should not blindly abandon conventional cancer treatment. For some cancers, there are very good chemotherapeutic, radiotherapeutic, or surgical treatments. For other forms of cancer, treatments are mediocre or poor. In addition, there are side effects to such treatments. One needs to consider the risk-benefit balance of utilizing these methods. I feel it would be tragic to pursue the healing of life-threatening disease without considering the medical treatments that are available. I also think it would be equally tragic to pursue conventional therapy without first considering the effectiveness of those treatments and their side effects as well as the complementary approaches that are available.

Conclusion

It is my hope that I have given a small glimpse of a few of the many ways I find macrobiotics and modern science to be consistent with each other. As more and more people learn about macrobiotics, both modern medicine and macrobiotics itself will continue to undergo change. Science will verify many more things that macrobiotics has been saying for years. At some point I believe both perspectives will reach similar conclusions. The truth will ultimately withstand the scrutiny of both perspectives. When the Eastern and Western perspectives come together it is my belief that we will begin to solve a great deal of today's health problems.

References

[1] Philips, F., 'Isocaloric Diet Changes and Electroencephalographic Sleep," *Lancet* 2 (1975): 723.

[2] Hippocrates, "On Airs, Waters and Places," translated and republished in *Medical Classics*, 3: 19–42, 1938.

[3] *Journal of American Dietetic Association*, 67: 455–59.

[4] Munro, H. N., *Annual Review of Nutrition*. 6: 1–12, 1986.

[5] Ibid., p. 5

[6] United States Senate Select Committee on Nutrition and Human Needs, *Dietary Goals for the United States*, 1977, (Revised 1980.)

[7] Ibid.

[8] *New England Journal of Medicine*, 292: 1148–51, 1975.

[9] Fraser, G., *American Journal of Clinical Nutrition*, 34: 1272, 1981.

[10] Caroll, K., *Cancer Research*, 35: 3374, 1975.

[11] Willett, W. C. and MacMahon, B., "Diet and Cancer—An Overview," *New England Journal of Medicine*, 310: 633–638, 1984.

[12] *JNCI*, Vol. 75, 1: 37, July 1985.

Appendix A:

Standard Dietary and Way of Life Suggestions

Daily Dietary Recommendations*

1. Whole Cereal Grains. At least 50 percent by volume of every meal is recommended to include cooked, organically grown, whole cereal grains prepared in a variety of ways. Whole cereal grains include brown rice, barley, millet, oats, corn, rye, wheat, and buckwheat. Please note that a small portion of this amount may consist of noodles or pasta, unyeasted whole grain breads, and other partially processed whole cereal grains.

2. Soups. Approximately 5 to 10 percent of your daily food intake may include soup made with vegetables, sea vegetables (wakame or kombu), grains or beans. Seasonings are usually miso or tamari soy sauce. The flavor should not be too salty.

3. Vegetables. About 20 to 30 percent of daily intake may include local and organically grown vegetables. Preferably, the majority are cooked in various styles (e.g. sautéed with a small amount of sesame or corn oil, steamed, boiled and sometimes prepared using tamari soy sauce or light sea salt as a seasoning). A small portion may be eaten as raw salad. Pickled vegetables without spice may also be used daily in small volume.

Vegetables for daily use include green cabbage, kale, broccoli, cauliflower, collards, pumpkin, watercress, Chinese cabbage, bok choy, dandelion, mustard greens, daikon greens, scallion, onions, daikon, turnips, acorn squash, butternut squash, buttercup squash, burdock, carrots, and other seasonally available varieties.

---

* For persons living in a temperate climate.

Avoid potatoes (including sweet potatoes and yams), tomatoes, eggplant, peppers, asparagus, spinach, beets, zucchini, and avocado from regular use. Mayonnaise and other oily dressings should be avoided.

4. Beans and Sea Vegetables. Approximately 5 to 10 percent of our daily diet includes cooked beans and sea vegetables. The most suitable beans for regular use are azuki beans, chick-peas, and lentils. Other beans may be used on occasion. Bean products such as tofu, tempeh, and natto can also be used. Sea vegetables such as nori, wakame, kombu, hijiki, arame, dulse, agar-agar, and Irish moss my be prepared in a variety of ways. They can be cooked with beans or vegetables, used in soups, or served separately as side dishes, flavored with a moderate amount of tamari soy sauce, sea salt, brown rice vinegar, umeboshi plum, umeboshi vinegar, and others.

5. Occasional Foods. If needed or desired, 1 to 3 times a week, approximately 5 to 10 percent of that day's consumption of food can include fresh white-meat fish such as flounder, sole, cod, carp, halibut, or trout.

Fruit or fruit desserts, including fresh, dried, and cooked fruits, may also be served two or three times a week. Local and organically grown fruits are preferred. If you live in a temperate climate, avoid tropical and semi-tropical fruit and eat, instead, temperate-climate fruits such as apples, pears, plums, peaches, apricots, berries, and melons. Frequent use of fruit juice is not advisable. However, occasional consumption in warmer weather may be appropriate depending on your health.

Lightly roasted nuts and seeds such as pumpkin, sesame, and sunflower seeds, peanuts, walnuts, and pecans may be enjoyed as a snack.

Rice syrup, barley malt, *amazaké*, and mirin may be used as a sweetener; brown rice vinegar or umeboshi vinegar may be used occasionally for a sour taste.

6. Beverages. Recommended daily beverages include roasted bancha twig tea, stem tea, roasted brown rice tea, roasted barley tea, dandelion tea, and cereal grain coffee. Any traditional tea that does not have an aromatic fragrance or a stimulating effect can be used. You may also drink a moderate amount of water (preferably spring or well water of good quality) but not iced.

7. Foods to Avoid for Better Health. Meat, animal fat, eggs, poultry, dairy products (including butter, yogurt, ice cream, milk, and cheese), refined sugars, chocolate, molasses, honey, other simple sugars and foods treated with them, and vanilla.

Tropical or semi-tropical fruits and fruit juices, soda, artificial drinks and beverages, coffee, colored tea, and all aromatic stimulating teas such as mint or peppermint tea.

All artificially colored, preserved, sprayed, or chemically treated foods. All refined and polished grains, flours, and their derivatives. Mass-produced industrialized food including all canned, frozen, and irradiated foods. Hot spices, any aromatic, stimulating food or food accessory, artificial vinegar, and strong alcoholic beverages.

8. Additional Suggestions. Cooking oil should be vegetable quality only. To improve your health, it is preferable to use only unrefined sesame or corn oil in moderate amounts.

- Salt should be naturally processed sea salt. Traditional, non-chemicalized shoyu or tamari soy sauce and miso may also be used as seasonings.
- Recommendable condiments include:
  —Gomashio (12 to 18 parts roasted sesame seeds to 1 part roasted sea salt)
  —Sea vegetable powder (kelp, kombu, wakame, and other sea vegetables)
  —Sesame sea vegetable powder
  —Umeboshi plums
  —Tekka
  —Tamari soy sauce or shoyu (moderate use, use only in cooking for mild flavoring)
  —Pickles (made using bran, miso, tamari soy sauce, salt), sauerkraut

- Your may have meals regularly, 2 to 3 times per day, as much as you want, provided the proportion is correct and chewing is thorough. Avoid eating for approximately 3 hours before sleeping.
- Proper cooking is very important for health. Everyone should learn to cook either by attending classes or under the guidance of an experienced macrobiotic cook. The recipes included in macrobiotic cookbooks may also be used in planning your meals.

Special Advice:

- The guidelines presented above are general suggestions. These suggestions may require modification depending on your special condition. Of course, any serious condition should be closely monitored by the appropriate medical, nutritional, and health professional.
- Along with beginning to change your diet, we invite you to attend any of our regular study programs or seminars and to meet personally with a qualified macrobiotic teacher as well as attending cooking classes.

Way of Life Suggestions

- Live each day happily without being preoccupied with your health; try to keep mentally and physically active.
- View everything and everyone you meet with gratitude, particularly offering thanks before and after every meal.
- Please chew your food very well, at least 50 times per mouthful, or until it becomes liquid.
- It is best to avoid wearing synthetic or woolen clothes directly on the skin. As much as possible, wear cotton, especially for undergarments. Avoid excessive metallic accessories on the fingers, wrists, or neck. Keep such ornaments simple and graceful.
- If your strength permits, go outdoors in simple clothing. Walk on the grass, beach, or soil up to one-half hour every day. Keep

your home in good order, from the kitchen, bathroom, bedroom, and living rooms, to every corner of the house.

- Initiate and maintain an active correspondence, extending your best wishes to parents, children, brothers and sisters, teachers, and friends.
- Avoid taking long hot baths or showers unless you have been consuming too much salt or animal food.
- To increase circulation, scrub your entire body with a hot, damp towel every morning or every night. If that is not possible, at least scrub your hands, feet, fingers, and toes.
- Avoid chemically perfumed cosmetics. For care of the teeth, brush with natural preparations or sea salt.
- If your condition permits, exercise regularly as part of daily life, including activities like walking, scrubbing floors, cleaning windows, washing clothes and working in the garden. You may also participate in exercise programs such as yoga, martial arts, dance or sports.
- Avoid using electric cooking devices (ovens and ranges) or microwave ovens. Convert to gas or wood-stove cooking at the earliest opportunity.
- It is best to minimize the use of color television and computer display units.
- Include some large green plants in your house to freshen and enrich the oxygen content of the air of your home.
- Sing a happy song every day.

These guidelines are intended to supplement consultation with a medical or nutritional professional or personal guidance received from a qualified macrobiotic teacher.

We wish to express our gratitude and support to the following organizations for their dietary recommendations as expressed in their publications:

Dietary Goals for the United States, published in 1977 (revised in 1980) by the U. S. Senate Select Committee on Nutrition and Human Needs.

Healthy People: *Health Promotion and Disease Prevention*, published in 1979 by the U. S. Surgeon General.

Diet, Nutrition, and Cancer, published in 1982 by the National Academy of Sciences.

and to the reports and statements made by the:

• American Heart Association
• American Diabetes Association
• American Society for Clinical Nutrition
• American Cancer Society

For information on macrobiotic educational programs, call or write:

Kushi Institute
P. O. Box 1100, 17 Station St., Brookline, MA 02147
(617) 738–0045

Appendix B:

Classification of Yin and Yang

Characteristic	YIN (▽) Centrifugal Force	YANG (△) Centripetal Force
Tendency	Expansion	Contraction
Function	Diffusion	Fusion
	Dispersion	Assimilation
	Separation	Gathering
	Decomposition	Organization
Movement	More inactive and slower	More active and faster
Vibration	Shorter wave and higher frequency	Longer wave and lower frequency
Direction	Ascent and vertical	Descent and horizontal
Position	More outward and peripheral	More inward and central
Weight	Lighter	Heavier
Temperature	Colder	Hotter
Light	Darker	Brighter
Humidity	More wet	More dry
Density	Thinner	Thicker
Size	Longer	Smaller
Shape	More expansive and fragile	More contractive and harder
Form	Longer	Shorter
Texture	Softer	Harder
Atomic particle	Electron	Proton
Elements	N, O, K, P, Ca, etc.	H, C, Na, As, Mg, etc.
Environment	Vibration . . . Air . . . Water . . .	Earth
Climatic effects	Tropical climate	Colder climate
Biology	More vegetable quality	More animal quality
Sex	Female	Male
Organ structure	More hollow and expansive	More compacted and condensed
Nerves	More peripheral, orthosympathetic	More central, parasympathetic
Attitude	More gentle, negative	More active, positive
Work	More psychological and mental	More physical and social
Dimension	Space	Time

Notes on the Contributors

Henry Edward Altenberg, M.D. has practiced psychiatry for thirty-five years, and is certified by the American Board of Psychiatry and the American Board of Child Psychiatry. He has published occasional articles in *Voices*, the Journal of the American Academy of Psychotherapy, and currently practices in Kittery, Maine and Portsmouth, New Hampshire. Dr. Altenberg is married with four children.

Guillermo Asis, M.D. practices at Wellbeing Medical Associates in Brookline, Massachusetts. He has a general practice with an emphasis on internal medicine, cardiology, macrobiotics, and homeopathy.

Martha C. Cottrell, M.D. is in private practice in New York City specializing in health promotion and disease prevention. She is also a director of student health at one of the State Universities in New York City. She received her boards in family medicine in 1969, and is a graduate of Women's Medical College of Pennsylvania, class of '62, and a fellow in preventive and community medicine, New York City, 1981–82. She is a frequent lecturer on the need to emphasize prevention and health promotion in Western medicine.

For the past three years, Dr. Cottrell has been the clinical administrator and medical consultant for the AIDS research project in conjunction with the Boston University School of Medicine, Department of Microbiology, and the Kushi Foundation of Boston, studying the effects of macrobiotics as alternative and adjunctive therapy for AIDS. She is coauthor, with Michio Kushi, of *AIDS: Cause and Solution*, publsihed by Japan Publications and distributed by Haper and Row.

David Dodson, M.D. studied medicine at the University of Ottawa where he received his M.D. Following graduation he moved to Boston to pursue post graduate training at Harvard. He now practices in Boston where he specializes in internal medicine and nutrition.

Helen Farrell, M.D. is a graduate of the University of Ottawa Medical School. She underwent two years of surgical training and is a former medical consultant for the Department of National Health and Welfare in Canada. She is currently in general practice in Ottawa, specializing in PMS, menopause, and nutrition.

Stephen Harnish, M.D. is currently clinical director of supportive services for the outpatient department of the Mental Health Center of Greater Manchester, New Hampshire. He is a graduate of the University of New Mexico School of Medicine and the Dartmouth Medical School Psychiatry Program. He is former medical director of New Hampshire Hospital and has served in the New Hampshire state legislature.

Marc Van Cauwenberghe, M.D. received his medical degree from the University of Ghent in 1969. Soon after, he began the macrobiotic way of life, and in 1972, journeyed from his native Belgium to Boston to begin studies with Michio Kushi. Since then he has traveled and lectured extensively throughout Europe and the United States, and has coauthored several books, including *Natural Healing through Macrobiotics* and *Macrobiotic Home Remedies*. He is a member of the faculty of the Kushi Institute, and is currently working on a book featuring the essays of George Ohsawa.

Lawrence H. Kushi, Sc.D. is a nutritional epidemiologist at the cancer prevention research unit at the Fred Hutchinson Cancer Research Center in Seattle. He worked previously in the division of epidemiology at the University of Minnesota, and received his doctoral degree in nutrition at the Harvard School of Public Health. He has taught at the Kushi Institute and at other macrobiotic educational centers, and is currently working to apply research to further understanding of diet and health for the goal of world peace.

Vivien Newbold, M.D. received her medical training at the University of Edinburgh and went on to specialize in emergency medicine. In 1984 she became a fellow of the American College of Emergency Physicians, and practices as an emergency physician in Philadelphia. Since 1983 Dr. Newbold has been following the macrobiotic way of life, and sees patients who want to learn more about taking responsibility for their own life and health, and preventive medicine. She also lectures on macrobiotics, and gives healing massage.

Christiane Northrup, M.D. is a clinical assistant professor of obstetrics and gynecology at the University of Vermont. She is currently president of the American Holistic Medical Foundation and co-founder of *Women to Women*, an innovative women's health care center in Yarmouth, Maine. She is a frequent contributor to *East West Journal*, and a regular speaker at macrobiotic conferences and seminars. She is married with two daughters.

Terry Shintani, M.D. received degrees in medicine and law from the University of Hawaii, and an MPH in nutrition from Harvard University. He is currently in private practice in general and preventive medicine in Hawaii, with emphasis on nutrition related diseases, and is the coordinator of a clinic based preventive health program. He has been macrobiotic for more than twelve years and has studied at the Kushi Institute in Boston.

Macrobiotic Resources

● **Macrobiotic Way of Life Seminar**

The *Macrobiotic Way of Life Seminar* is an introductory program offered by the Kushi Institute in Boston. It includes classes in macrobiotic cooking, home care, and kitchen setup, lectures on the philosophy of macrobiotics and the standard diet, and individual way of life guidance. It is presented monthly and includes introductory and intermediate level programs. Information on the *Macrobiotic Way of Life Seminar* is available from:

> The Kushi Institute
> 17 Station Street
> Brookline, Massachusetts 02147
> (617) 738–0045

● **Macrobiotic Residential Seminar**

The *Macrobiotic Residential Seminar* is an introductory program offered at the Kushi Foundation Berkshires Center in Becket, Massachusetts. It is a one week live-in program that includes hands-on training in macrobiotic cooking and home care, lectures on the philosophy and practice of macrobiotics, and meals prepared by a specially trained cooking staff. It is presented monthly and includes introductory and intermediate levels. Information on the *Macrobiotic Residential Seminar* is available from:

> Kushi Foundation Berkshires Center
> Box 7
> Becket, Massachusetts 01223
> (413) 623–5742

● **Kushi Institute Leadership Studies**

For those who wish to study further, the Kushi Institute in Boston offers instruction for individuals who wish to become trained and certified macrobiotic teachers. Similar leadership training programs are offered at Kushi Institute affiliates in London, Amsterdam, Antwerp, Florence, as well as in Portugal and Switzerland. Information on *Leadership Studies* is available from the Kushi Institute in Boston.

• Other Programs

The Kushi Institute offers a variety of public programs including an annual Summer Conference in western Massachusetts, special weight-loss and natural beauty seminars, and intensive cooking and spiritual development training at the Berkshires Center. Information on these programs is available at either of the above addresses. Moreover, macrobiotic educational centers throughout the United States, Canada, and the world offer a variety of introductory and special programs. The Kushi Foundation publishes a *Worldwide Macrobiotic Directory* every year listing these centers and individuals. Please consult the *Directory* for the nearest macrobiotic center or qualified instructor.

• Publications

Books and publications with information on macrobiotics are available from the Kushi Foundation, or at other macrobiotic centers, natural foodstores, and bookstores. Ongoing developments are reported in the Kushi Foundation's periodicals, including the *East West Journal*, a monthly magazine begun in 1971 and now with an international readership of 200,000. The *EWJ* features regular articles on the macrobiotic approach to health and nutrition, as well as related subjects. Moreover, Michio and Aveline Kushi have authored numerous books on macrobiotic philosophy, cooking, diet, and way of life. The following titles are especially recommended for further study:

• Books by Michio Kushi

Health and Diet

1. *The Cancer-Prevention Diet* (with Alex Jack, St. Martin's Press, 1983)
2. *Diet for a Strong Heart* (with Alex Jack, St. Martin's Press, 1985)
3. *Natural Healing through Macrobiotics* (edited by Edward Esko and Marc Van Cauwenberghe, MD, Japan Publications, 1979)
4. *Macrobiotic Home Remedies* (edited by Marc Van Cauwenberghe, MD, Japan Publications, 1985)
5. *Macrobiotic Diet* (co-authored with Aveline Kushi; edited by Alex Jack, Japan Publications, 1985)
6. *Cancer and Heart Disease: The Macrobiotic Approach* (with various contributors; edited by Edward Esko, Japan Publications, 1982)
7. *Crime and Diet: The Macrobiotic Approach* (with various contributors; edited by Edward Esko, Japan Publications, 1987)

8. *AIDS: Cause and Solution—The Macrobiotic Approach to Natural Immunity* (co-authored with Martha C. Cottrell, MD, Japan Publications, 1988)

9. *Macrobiotic Health Education Series—Diabetes and Hypogylcemia; Allergies; Obesity, Weight Loss and Eating Disorders; Infertility and Reproductive Disorders; Arthritis; Stress and Hypertension* (with various editors, Japan Publications, 1985–88)

10. *How to See Your Health: the Book of Oriental Diagnosis* (Japan Publications, 1980)

11. *Your Face Never Lies* (Avery Publishing Group, 1983)

Philosophy and Way of Life

1. *One Peaceful World* (with Alex Jack, St. Martin's Press, 1986)

2. *The Book of Macrobiotics: The Universal Way of Health, Happiness, and Peace* (with Alex Jack, Japan Publications, revised edition, 1986)

3. *The Macrobiotic Way* (with Stephen Blauer, Avery Publishing Group, 1985)

4. *The Book of Do-In* (Japan Publications, 1979)

5. *Macrobiotic Palm Healing* (with Olivia Oredson Saunders, Japan Publications, 1988)

6. *On the Greater View* (Avery Publishing Group, 1986)

● **Books by Aveline Kushi**

Cooking

1. *Aveline Kushi's Complete Guide to Macrobiotic Cooking for Health, Harmony, and Peace* (with Alex Jack, Warner Books, 1985)

2. *Aveline Kushi's Introducing Macrobiotic Cooking* (with Wendy Esko, Japan Publications, 1987)

3. *The Changing Seasons Macrobiotic Cookbook* (with Wendy Esko, Avery Publishing Group, 1985)

4. *How to Cook with Miso* (Japan Publications, 1979)

5. *Macrobiotic Family Favorites* (with Wendy Esko, Japan Publications, 1987)

6. *The Macrobiotic Cancer Prevention Cookbook* (with Wendy Esko, Avery Publishing Group, 1988)

7. *Macrobiotic Food and Cooking Series—Diabetes and Hypogylcemia; Allergies; Obesity, Weight Loss and Eating Disorders; Infertility*

and Reproductive Disorders; Arthritis; Stress and Hypertension (with various editors, Japan Publications, 1985–88)

Family Health

1. *Macrobiotic Pregnancy and Care of the Newborn* (with Michio Kushi; edited by Edward and Wendy Esko, Japan Publications, 1984)
2. *Macrobiotic Child Care and Family Health* (with Michio Kushi; edited by Edward and Wendy Esko, Japan Publications, 1986)
3. *Lessons of Night and Day* (Avery Publishing Group, 1985)

Philosophy and Way of Life

1. *Aveline: The Life and Dream of the Woman Behind Macrobiotics Today* (with Alex Jack, Japan Publications, 1988)

In addition, macrobiotic publications by various authors are listed in the bibliography. These are also recommended for further study.

Recommended Reading

Books

Aihara, Cornellia: *The Dō of Cooking*. Chico, Calif.: George Ohsawa Macrobiotic Foundation, 1972.

———. *Macrobiotic Childcare*. Oroville, Calif.: George Ohsawa Macrobiotic Foundation, 1971.

———. *Macrobiotic Kitchen: Key to Good Health*. Tokyo & New York: Japan Publications, Inc., 1982.

Aihara, Herman. *Basic Macrobiotics*. Tokyo & New York: Japan Publications, Inc., 1985.

Benedict, Dirk. *Confessions of a Kamikaze Cowboy*. Van Nuys, Calif.: Newcastle, 1987.

Brown, Virginia, with Susan Stayman. *Macrobiotic Miracle: How a Vermont Family Overcame Cancer*. Tokyo & New York: Japan Publications, Inc., 1985.

Dietary Goals for the United States. Washington, D. C.: Select Committee on Nutrition and Human Needs, U.S. Senate, 1977.

Diet, Nutrition, and Cancer. Washington, D. C.: National Academy of Sciences, 1982.

Dufty, William. *Sugar Blues*. New York: Warner Books, 1975.

Esko, Wendy. *Aveline Kushi's Introducing Macrobiotic Cooking*. Tokyo & New York: Japan Publications, Inc., 1987.

Esko, Edward and Wendy. *Macrobiotic Cooking for Everyone*. Tokyo & New York: Japan Publications, Inc., 1980.

Esko, Edward, ed. *Doctors Look at Macrobiotics*. Tokyo & New York: Japan Publications, Inc., 1988.

Fukuoka, Masanobu. *The Natural Way of Farming*. Tokyo & New York: Japan Publications, Inc., 1985.

———. *The Road Back to Nature*. Tokyo & New York: Japan Publications, Inc., 1987.

———. *The One-Straw Revolution*. Emmaus, Pa.: Rodale Press, 1978.

Healthy People: The Surgeon General's Report on Health Promotion and Disease Prevention, Washington, D. C.: Government Printing Office, 1979.

Heidenry, Carolyn. *Making the Transition to a Macrobiotic Diet*. Wayne, N.J.: Avery Publishing Group, 1987.

Hippocrates. *Hippocratic Writings*. Edited by G. E. R. Lloyd. Translated by J. Chadwick and W. N. Mann. New York: Penguin Books, 1978.

I Ching or Book of Changes. Translated by Richard Wilhelm and Cary F. Baynes. Princeton: Bollingen Foundation, 1950.

Ineson, John. *The Way of Life: Macrobiotics and the Spirit of Christianity.* Tokyo & New York: Japan Publications, Inc., 1986.

Ishida, Eiwan. *Genmai: Brown Rice for Better Health.* Tokyo & New York: Japan Publications, Inc., 1988.

Jack, Gale with Alex Jack. *Promenade Home: Macrobiotics and Women's Health.* Tokyo & New York: Japan Publications, Inc., 1988.

Jacobs, Barbara and Leonard. *Cooking with Seitan: The Delicious Natural Food from Whole Grain.* Tokyo & New York: Japan Publications, Inc., 1986.

Jacobson, Michael. *The Changing American Diet.* Washington, D. C.: Center for Science in the Public Interest, 1978.

Kaibara, Ekiken. *Yojokun: Japanese Secrets of Good Health.* Tokyo: Tokuma Shoten, 1974.

Kidder, Ralph D. and Edward F. Kelly. *Choice for Survival: The Baby Boomer's Dilemma.* Tokyo & New York: Japan Pbulications, Inc., 1988.

Kohler, Jean and Mary Alice. *Healing Miracles from Macrobiotics.* West Nyack, N. Y.: Parker, 1979.

Kotzsch, Ronald. *Macrobiotics: Yesterday and Today.* Tokyo & New York: Japan Publications, Inc., 1985.

———. *Macrobiotics Beyond Food.* Tokyo & New York: Japan Publications, Inc., 1988.

Kushi, Aveline. *How to Cook with Miso.* Tokyo & New York: Japan Publications, Inc., 1978.

———. *Lessons of Night and Day.* Wayne, New Jersey: Avery Publishing Group, 1985.

———. *Macrobiotic Food and Cooking Series: Diabetes and Hypoglycemia; Allergies.* Tokyo & New York: Japan Publications, Inc., 1985.

———. *Macrobiotic Food and Cooking Series: Obesity, Weight Loss, and Eating Disorders; Infertility and Reproductive Disorders.* Tokyo & New York: Japan Publications, Inc., 1987.

Kushi, Aveline, with Alex Jack. *Aveline Kushi's Complete Guide to Macrobiotic Cooking.* New York: Warner Books, 1985.

———. *Aveline: The Life and Dream of the Woman Behind Macrobiotics Today.* Tokyo & New York: Japan Publications, Inc., 1988.

Kushi, Aveline and Michio. *Macrobiotic Pregnancy and Care of the*

Newborn. Edited by Edward and Wendy Esko. Tokyo & New York: Japan Publications, Inc., 1984.

———. *Macrobiotic Child Care and Family Health.* Tokyo & New York: Japan Publications, Inc., 1986.

Kushi, Aveline, and Wendy Esko. *Macrobiotic Family Favorites.* Tokyo & New York: Japan Publications, Inc., 1987.

Kushi, Aveline, and Wendy Esko. *The Changing Seasons Macrobiotic Cookbook.* Wayne, N. J.: Avery Publishing Group, 1983.

———. *The Macrobiotic Cancer Prevention Cookbook.* Wayne, New Jersey: Avery Publishing Group, 1986.

Kushi, Michio. *The Book of Dō-In: Exercise for Physical and Spiritual Development.* Tokyo & New York: Japan Publications, Inc., 1979.

———. *The Book of Macrobiotics: The Universal Way of Health, Happiness and Peace.* Tokyo & New York: Japan Publications, Inc., 1986 (Rev. ed.).

———. *Cancer and Heart Disease: The Macrobiotic Approach to Degenerative Disorders.* Tokyo & New York: Japan Publications, Inc., 1986 (Rev. ed.).

———. *Crime and Diet: The Macrobiotic Approach.* Tokyo & New York: Japan Publications, Inc., 1987.

———. *The Era of Humanity.* Brookline, Mass.: East West Journal, 1980.

———. *How to See Your Health: The Book of Oriental Diagnosis.* Tokyo & New York: Japan Publications, Inc., 1980.

———. *Macrobiotic Health Education Series: Diabetes and Hypoglycemia; Allergies.* Tokyo & New York: Japan Publications, Inc., 1985.

———. *Macrobiotic Health Education Series: Obesity, Weight Loss, and Eating Disorders; Infertility and Reproductive Disorders.* Tokyo & New York: Japan Publications, Inc., 1987.

———. *Natural Healing through Macrobiotics.* Tokyo & New York: Japan Publications, Inc., 1978.

———. *On the Greater View: Collected Thoughts on Macrobiotics and Humanity.* Wayne, New Jersey: Avery Publishing Group, 1985.

———. *Your Face Never Lies.* Wayne, N. J.: Avery Publishing Group, 1983.

Kushi, Michio, and Alex Jack. *The Cancer-Prevention Diet.* New York: St. Martin's Press, 1983.

———. *Diet for a Strong Heart.* New York: St. Martin's Press, 1984.

Kushi, Michio, with Alex Jack. *One Peaceful World.* New York: St. Martin's Press, 1987.

Kushi, Michio and Aveline, with. Alex Jack. *The Macrobiotic Die* Tokyo & New York: Japan Publications, Inc., 1985.

Kushi, Michio and Martha C. Cottrell. *AIDS: Cause and Solution— The Macrobiotic Approach to Natural Immunity.* Tokyo & New York Japan Publications, Inc., 1988.

Kushi, Michio, and the East West Foundation. *The Macrobiotic Ap proach to Cancer.* Wayne, N. J.: Avery Publishing Group, 1982.

Kushi, Michio, with Stephen Blauer. *The Macrobiotic Way.* Wayn• New Jersey: Avery Publishing Group, 1985.

Kushi, Michio with Olivia Oredson. *Macrobiotic Palm Healing: Energ at Your Finger-tips.* Tokyo & New York: Japan Publications, Inc. 1988.

Levin, Cecile Tovah. *Cooking for Regeneration: Macrobiotic Relie from Cancer, AIDS, and Degenerative Disease.* Tokyo & New York Japan Publications, Inc., 1988.

Mendelsohn, Robert S., M.D. *Confessions of a Medical Heretic* Chicago: Contemporary Books, 1979.

———. *Male Practice.* Chicago: Contemporary Books, 1980.

Nussbaum, Elaine. *Recovery: From Cancer to Health through Macro biotics.* Tokyo & New York: Japan Publications, Inc., 1986.

Nutrition and Mental Health. Washington, D. C.: Select Committee on Nutrition and Human Needs, U.S. Senate, 1977, 1980.

Ohsawa, George, *Cancer and the Philosophy of the Far East.* Oroville, Calif.: George Ohsawa Macrobiotic Foundation, 1971 edition.

———. *You Are All Sanpaku.* Edited by William Dufty, New York: University Books, 1965.

———. *Zen Macrobiotics.* Los Angeles: Ohsawa Foundation, 1965.

Ohsawa, Lima. *Macrobiotic Cuisine.* Tokyo & New York: Japan Publications, Inc., 1984.

Polatin, Betsy. *Macrobiotics in Motion: Yin and Yang in Moving Spirals.* Tokyo & New York: Japan Publications, Inc., 1987.

Price, Western, A., D.D.S. *Nutrition and Physical Degeneration.* Santa Monica, Calif.: Price-Pottenger Nutritional Foundation, 1945.

Sattilaro, Anthony, M.D., with Tom Monte. *Recalled by Life: The Story of My Recovery from Cancer.* Boston: Houghton-Mifflin, 1982.

Schauss, Alexander. *Diet, Crime, and Delinquency.* Berkeley, Calif.: Parker House, 1980.

Scott, Neil E., with Jean Farmer. *Eating with Angels.* Tokyo & New York: Japan Publications, Inc., 1986.

Sergel, David. *The Macrobiotic Way of Zen Shiatsu.* Tokyo & New York: Japan Publications, Inc., 1988.

Tara, William. *A Challenge to Medicine.* Tokyo & New York: Japan Publications, Inc., 1988.

———. *Macrobiotics and Human Behavior.* Tokyo & New York: Japan Publications, Inc., 1985.

Wood, Rebecca. *Quinoa the Supergrain: Ancient Food for Today.* Tokyo & New York: Japan Publications, Inc., 1988.

Yamamoto, Shizuko. *Barefoot Shiatsu.* Tokyo & New York: Japan Publications, Inc., 1979.

The Yellow Emperor's Classic of Internal Medicine. Translated by Ilza Veith, Berkeley: University of California Press, 1949.

Periodicals

East West Journal. Brookline, Mass.

Macromuse. Washington, D. C.

Nutrition Action. Washington, D. C.

"The People's Doctor" by Robert S. Mendelsohn, M.D. and Marian Tompson, Evanston, Ill.

Index